Perioperative Care of Cardiac Surgery Patients

Elsayed Elmistekawy • Nabil A. Shallik
Editors

Perioperative Care of Cardiac Surgery Patients

Springer

Editors
Elsayed Elmistekawy
Cardiac Surgery Division, Department of Surgery
University of Ottawa
Ottawa, ON, Canada

Nabil A. Shallik
Clinical Anaesthesiology Department
College of Medicine Qatar University and Weill Cornell Medical College
Doha, Qatar

ISBN 978-3-032-09816-0 ISBN 978-3-032-09817-7 (eBook)
https://doi.org/10.1007/978-3-032-09817-7

This Springer imprint is published by the registered company Springer Nature Switzerland AG
The registered company address is: Gewerbestrasse 11, 6330 Cham, Switzerland

Contents

Introduction

Elsayed Elmistekawy and Nabil A. Shallik

Care of adult cardiac surgery patients outside the operative room is one of the key elements for achieving excellent outcomes of cardiac surgery.

It starts before surgery begins with good planning on the timing and optimization of a patient's general and cardiac condition, continues to the immediate postsurgery period in the intensive care unit (ICU), and finally extends to the surgical stepdown units or the surgical ward.

The surgical ward is the largest hospital unit hosting all surgical patients before and after surgery.

Care of cardiac surgery patients in cardiac surgery wards is an important element of patient care, education, and interdisciplinary communication, and it is beneficial for general outcomes after surgery and patient satisfaction.

Despite being a key component of cardiac surgery patient care, the surgery ward does not receive the amount of attention that is devoted to care in the operative room or ICUs.

This book's main focus is to describe patient care in surgical wards; it is also intended to serve as a quick guide for clinicians responsible for patient care in surgical wards.

It will also help inform general practitioners, nurses, and medical students involved in the care of cardiac surgery patients.

Cardiac surgery patient care in surgical wards starts at the moment of admission, when it is crucial to assess and understand what a patient's needs and prepare the patient for the upcoming surgery.

E. Elmistekawy
Cardiac Surgery Division, Department of Surgery, University of Ottawa, Ottawa, ON, Canada

N. A. Shallik (✉)
Clinical Anaesthesiology Department, College of Medicine Qatar University and Weill Cornell Medical College, Doha, Qatar
e-mail: Nshallik@hamad.qa; nshallik@outlook.com

E. Elmistekawy, N. A. Shallik (eds.), *Perioperative Care of Cardiac Surgery Patients*, https://doi.org/10.1007/978-3-032-09817-7_1

Another important moment in patient care is the patient's transfer from the surgical ICU, a careful review of the surgery performed, the course of surgery, complications or concerns during surgery, drains, pacing wires, plan of staged surgery or intervention, and instructions for postoperative care.

The few days following surgery are very dynamic, with a long list of issues that not only affect a patient's cardiac status but also include all other body systems affected by the course of the initial disease and comorbidities, as well as the surgery performed and the path of the recovery period immediately following surgery.

Preparing the patient to transit from being a hospitalized patient to discharge is also very important and serves as an educational moment for patients and their families that can facilitate a smooth and full recovery, a return to normal life after surgery, and decreased risk of readmission. The for discharge plan should start when surgery is scheduled and be revisited after the operation is complete to address any new complications that might have arisen with the patient following discharge from the hospital.

This book is a brief and simple guide for clinicians caring for cardiac surgery patients on a surgical ward. It is meant to complement standard textbooks and teaching manuals dealing with cardiac surgery patient care. It is a kind of how-to manual summarizing the knowledge and skills management needs in connection with issues and complications faced by cardiac surgery patients on surgical wards.

Preoperative Management of Cardiac Surgical Patients

Bassam Shoman and Sameh Ramadan Aboulnaga

1 Introduction

Patients scheduled for cardiac surgery represent a distinct and high-risk population, often characterized by multiple comorbidities that may significantly influence both their perioperative course and overall hospital outcomes. Common comorbid conditions include long-standing hypertension, heart failure (HF), acute coronary syndrome (ACS), cardiomyopathy, severe valvular heart disease, clinically significant arrhythmias, peripheral vascular disease, thoracic aortic atheroma, insulin-dependent diabetes mellitus, renal insufficiency, chronic pulmonary disease, neurological disorders, anemia, and a history of prior cardiac surgery [1, 2].

A substantial proportion of these patients present for surgery under *urgent or emergent circumstances*, dictated by the severity or acuteness of their underlying cardiac pathology. In some cases, surgery is performed as a *salvage procedure*—for example, in patients diagnosed with critical coronary artery disease during coronary angiography in the catheterization laboratory, or in those with life-threatening, rapidly progressive conditions such as acute aortic dissection. Similarly, acute valvular lesions, such as ischemic rupture of the papillary muscle resulting in severe, acute mitral regurgitation, may necessitate *emergency surgical intervention*.

In this chapter, we will focus on the *preoperative assessment* of patients undergoing cardiac surgery, with the aim of optimizing anesthetic management and improving perioperative outcomes [1].

B. Shoman (✉) · S. R. Aboulnaga
Hamad Medical Corporation, Heart Hospital, Doha, Qatar
e-mail: bshoman@hamad.qa; SAboulnaga@hamad.qa

E. Elmistekawy, N. A. Shallik (eds.), *Perioperative Care of Cardiac Surgery Patients*, https://doi.org/10.1007/978-3-032-09817-7_2

2 Multidisciplinary Team (MDT) Approach

Most cardiac centers maintain specialized anesthesia teams responsible not only for intraoperative anesthetic care but also for postoperative management in the surgical intensive care unit. The management of patients undergoing cardiac surgery should consistently be guided by a *multidisciplinary team (MDT) approach.*

An essential component of this approach is the establishment of a dedicated *pre-operative anesthesia clinic*, where elective surgical patients can undergo evaluation and any necessary investigations before hospital admission. This strategy reduces preoperative hospital stay, thereby minimizing the risk of hospital-acquired infections. To further streamline care, preadmission surgical and anesthesia clinic visits may be coordinated on the same day, expediting the surgical pathway and avoiding unnecessary procedural delays [3].

Weekly *joint conferences* involving both surgical and anesthesiology teams are recommended to review all patients scheduled for surgery in the upcoming week. These meetings facilitate *risk stratification*, comprehensive assessment of comorbidities, and the integration of multidisciplinary expertise. In addition to clinical history, prior investigations—including chest radiography, coronary angiography, and echocardiography—are systematically reviewed. Abnormal laboratory findings can be evaluated, and further consultations with relevant medical specialties arranged in advance of the planned procedure. Ultimately, *case scheduling* is determined by the urgency of the condition and the severity of the underlying disease [4].

3 Preoperative Assessment

The primary objective of preoperative assessment in patients undergoing cardiac surgery is the *optimization of their medical condition* prior to the procedure, as well as the *stratification of perioperative risk.* This process enables the anesthesiology team to formulate a tailored anesthetic and perioperative management plan, consistent with the most recent evidence-based guidelines.

Equally important, the preanesthetic consultation provides an opportunity to establish *patient rapport* and to mitigate *anxiety related to the surgical experience*, thereby improving patient cooperation and overall perioperative care.

The core components of preoperative assessment include:

1. *Comprehensive history taking*
2. *Detailed physical examination*
3. *Review of investigations and laboratory results*

3.1 Comprehensive History Taking

Before initiating history taking and preoperative assessment, it is essential to establish *patient rapport.* The anesthesiologist should explain their role in the perioperative management team, outline the anesthetic plan, and prepare the patient for the expected immediate postoperative course in the intensive care unit (ICU). Such communication is crucial to alleviate anxiety and facilitate smoother recovery [5].

3.1.1 Cardinal Symptoms of Cardiac Disease

The principal presenting symptoms in cardiac surgical patients include:

- *Chest pain/angina*
- *Palpitations*
- *Dyspnea/shortness of breath*
- *Reduced exercise tolerance*

Each symptom must be graded in terms of severity, patient tolerance, and the extent of limitation imposed on physical activity.

3.1.2 Angina and Ischemic Heart Disease

Myocardial ischemia typically presents as retrosternal, stabbing chest pain radiating to the left arm, neck, epigastrium, or back. The severity of angina can be classified using the *Canadian Cardiovascular Society (CCS) grading system* [6]:

- *Class I*: Angina only during strenuous, rapid, or prolonged exertion.
- *Class II*: Slight limitation of ordinary activity; symptoms triggered by walking uphill, emotional stress, or postprandial exertion.
- *Class III*: Marked limitation of ordinary activity; symptoms with walking 1–2 blocks or climbing one flight of stairs.
- *Class IV*: Inability to perform any activity without angina; symptoms may occur at rest.

Increasing severity of angina correlates with higher operative urgency and elevated risk of perioperative ischemia and postoperative complications.

Risk categories include:

- *Minimal risk*: No myocardial infarction (MI) or hemodynamic instability → elective surgery.
- *Intermediate risk*: MI without hemodynamic instability; managed with antiplatelets and low-molecular-weight heparin → urgent surgery.
- *High risk*: Ongoing ischemia/MI with hemodynamic compromise → emergency revascularization indicated.

3.1.3 Cardiac History and Prior Admissions

Patients often present with prior hospitalizations for decompensated cardiac conditions or procedures such as coronary angiography. A detailed review of each admission is necessary to identify complications or disease progression [7].

Frequent admissions for *decompensated heart failure (HF)* are associated with increased perioperative morbidity and mortality. Clinical features include exertional or resting dyspnea, orthopnea, palpitations, pedal edema, and pulmonary edema with productive cough or hemoptysis [8, 9].

Functional status should be categorized using the *New York Heart Association (NYHA) classification* [10]:

- *Class I*: No limitation of physical activity.
- *Class II*: Slight limitation; ordinary activity causes symptoms ("mild HF").
- *Class III*: Marked limitation; symptoms with less than ordinary activity ("moderate HF").
- *Class IV*: Symptoms at rest; any activity worsens discomfort ("severe HF").

3.1.4 Neurological Considerations

Patients with a history of *stroke or transient ischemic attack (TIA)* require thorough neurological evaluation to identify residual deficits. Hemodynamic variability during surgery may adversely impact neurological outcomes.

3.1.5 Renal Function

Preoperative renal insufficiency is common in cardiac patients, often secondary to chronic HF or contrast exposure during angiography. It increases the risk of postoperative morbidity and mortality. Cardiac surgery itself predisposes to *acute kidney injury (AKI)* due to aortic cross-clamping, fluctuating hemodynamics, use of blood products, and vasopressors. A history of dialysis or renal replacement therapy must be noted, and *arteriovenous fistula sites should be carefully documented and protected* from cannulation [11, 12].

3.1.6 Vascular and Atherosclerotic Disease

Atherosclerosis frequently coexists with coronary artery disease, particularly in patients with diabetes mellitus. Routine *carotid Doppler ultrasound* is indicated prior to elective or urgent cardiac surgery in patients >65 years or those with a history of stroke or TIA [13].

3.1.7 Arrhythmias and Device Therapy

Palpitations are common in valvular and ischemic heart disease. Preoperative medications, such as beta-blockers and amiodarone, should be reviewed. Malignant arrhythmias may present intraoperatively. Patients with implanted *pacemakers or implantable cardioverter-defibrillators (ICDs)* require device interrogation and reprogramming by the electrophysiology team prior to induction to avoid interference from electrocautery [1].

3.1.8 Lifestyle and Special Considerations

- *Smoking and alcohol use* should be assessed, as withdrawal syndromes may complicate postoperative recovery.
- *Pulmonary and renal symptoms* should be thoroughly evaluated.

- Patients with prior *gastric surgery* or *mediastinal radiation* should be screened for contraindications to intraoperative transesophageal echocardiography (TEE) [14].
- *Drug and food allergies* must be clearly documented and flagged in the patient record.

3.1.9 Endocrine Disorders

Diabetes mellitus must be carefully assessed, with documentation of:

- Type of diabetes (nondiabetic, diet-controlled, oral therapy, insulin-dependent)
- Duration of disease and treatment regimen
- Glycemic control (HbA1c, fasting blood glucose)

3.2 Physical Examination

A meticulous physical examination is a fundamental component of preoperative evaluation, providing crucial information for anesthetic and surgical planning.

3.2.1 General Examination

The initial assessment should include evaluation of the patient's *neurological status* to detect any residual deficits from prior ischemic or embolic stroke [15]. This is particularly important as perioperative hemodynamic fluctuations may exacerbate neurological compromise.

3.2.2 Vital Signs

Vital signs must be carefully documented during the preanesthetic visit, with review of inpatient records when available. Particular attention should be given to:

- *Blood pressure*: Should be measured in both supine and sitting positions to detect postural hypotension, which may result from β-blocker therapy or hypovolemia. Bilateral measurements are recommended; any significant discrepancy warrants further investigation for possible vascular pathology.
- *Heart rate and rhythm*: Assessment for bradycardia, tachycardia, or irregular rhythm.

3.2.3 Peripheral Pulses

Palpation of peripheral pulses in both upper and lower limbs is essential to assess rate, volume, regularity, and symmetry. In some patients, the *radial artery* may have been previously utilized for coronary angiography; a feeble pulse or local inflammation on that side indicates it should not be used for invasive arterial monitoring.

If the radial artery is considered as a potential graft, an *Allen test* should be performed on the nondominant hand to confirm ulnar collateral circulation (see Table 1).

Table 1 Allen test for assessment of ulnar collateral circulation [16]

Aspect	Standard Allen test	Modified Allen test
Purpose	Assess adequacy of ulnar collateral circulation before radial artery harvesting for CABG	Same purpose, but provides a more objective assessment
Equipment	None	Pulse oximeter
Procedure	1. Elevate hand, patient clenches fist for ~30 s. 2. Compress radial and ulnar arteries. 3. Patient opens/closes fist, hand appears blanched. 4. Release ulnar compression while maintaining radial compression.	1. Place pulse oximeter on thumb; record baseline saturation & waveform. 2. Compress radial & ulnar arteries until waveform disappears and SpO_2 drops. 3. Release ulnar artery compression.
Normal result	Palm flushes and color returns within 3–5 s → adequate ulnar collateral flow	Restoration of baseline waveform and oxygen saturation → adequate ulnar collateral flow
Abnormal result	Delayed (>5 s) or absent color return → inadequate ulnar collateral flow, radial harvest unsafe	Failure of waveform/saturation to recover → inadequate ulnar collateral flow

3.2.4 Cardiopulmonary Examination

- *Respiratory system*: Auscultation of both anterior and posterior lung fields should be performed to identify added sounds such as wheezes or crepitations, which may indicate pulmonary congestion or underlying chronic lung disease.
- *Cardiovascular system*: Cardiac auscultation may reveal rhythm irregularities, murmurs suggestive of valvular pathology, or additional abnormal heart sounds.

3.2.5 Neck and Airway Assessment

- *Neck examination*: Evaluation of the jugular venous landmarks is important for anticipating potential difficulties in central venous cannulation.
- *Airway evaluation*: Standard airway assessment, including documentation of the *Mallampati classification*, is necessary to predict intubation challenges. Patients with removable dentures should be advised to remove them prior to transfer to the operating theatre.

3.2.6 Patient Counseling and Consent

At the conclusion of the preanesthetic visit, the anesthesiologist should provide *patient education* regarding the anesthesia and surgical course. After discussion with the patient and family, a formal *informed anesthesia consent* must be obtained [17].

3.2.7 Functional Capacity Assessment

In high-risk patients, particularly those with *decompensated heart failure*, further objective evaluation of cardiorespiratory reserve may be warranted. Simple, inexpensive tools such as the *6-min walk test (6MWT)* and *incremental shuttle walk test* have been validated as predictors of favorable postoperative outcomes, although precise thresholds for early complication prediction require further evidence [18].

3.2.8 Extremity Examination

- *Upper limbs*: Assess radial and ulnar pulses, note handedness, evaluate for prior radial artery use in angiography, and perform Allen's test if radial grafting is anticipated.
- *Lower limbs*: Examine for edema, varicose veins (best assessed in the standing position), surgical scars, and integrity of peripheral pulses.

3.3 Laboratory and Diagnostic Investigations

A comprehensive review of laboratory and imaging investigations is an integral component of the preoperative assessment for cardiac surgery. These results provide essential guidance for risk stratification, perioperative optimization, and individualized anesthetic planning.

3.3.1 Hematology

- *Complete blood count (CBC)*:
  Hemoglobin levels must be reviewed to exclude anemia.
  - Anemia is defined as *Hb ≤ 13 g/dL in men* and *≤ 12 g/dL in women.*
  - Chronic anemia with positive fecal occult blood warrants gastroenterology evaluation to exclude *peptic ulcer disease* or *erosive gastritis.*
  - Correction should be achieved preoperatively with *oral or intravenous iron supplementation* and, when indicated, *erythropoietin therapy*, to minimize intraoperative transfusion requirements [19].
- *Platelet count and function*:
  Must be assessed to exclude *heparin-induced thrombocytopenia (HIT)* in patients exposed to heparin during coronary care unit (CCU) admission. Point-of-care platelet function assays are often available in cardiac centers and allow rapid decision-making regarding the need for platelet or factor transfusion in intraoperative coagulopathy.
- *Sickle cell screening* is mandatory for patients with a family history of sickle cell disease, and for individuals of *African, Mediterranean, East Indian, or Central American origin*, as perioperative hypoxemia and ischemia may precipitate vaso-occlusive crises.

3.3.2 Cardiac Biomarkers

- *Cardiac enzymes* provide an index of myocardial ischemia.
- *B-type natriuretic peptide (BNP)* reflects myocardial reserve and the severity of heart failure.

3.3.3 Renal Function

Renal function is best assessed using *creatinine clearance* rather than serum creatinine or blood urea nitrogen.

- *End-stage renal disease (ESRD)*: Patients should undergo *hemodialysis the day before surgery*, with frequent postoperative monitoring of serum electrolytes.
- *Ultrafiltration dialysis* may be considered during cardiopulmonary bypass for volume management in these patients.

3.3.4 Hepatic Function

Liver function tests should be reviewed, particularly in patients with *right-sided heart failure*, where hepatic congestion may impair perioperative metabolic reserve.

3.3.5 Endocrine Profile

- *HbA1c* measurement is essential in diabetic patients to assess long-term glycemic control.
- Strict *intraoperative glucose control protocols* reduce morbidity and the risk of surgical site infections.

3.3.6 Radiographic Imaging

- *Chest radiograph*: Provides a baseline for comparison in the perioperative period.
- *Carotid Doppler ultrasound*: Recommended in patients >65 years and those with severe CAD or left main coronary stenosis [1, 13].
  - If critical carotid stenosis with prior TIA/stroke is detected, referral to vascular surgery is warranted to determine the need for *concomitant carotid endarterectomy* or staged intervention.

3.3.7 Pulmonary Function Testing

Indicated in patients with *severe respiratory symptoms* or abnormal chest radiographs:

- *FEV_1 < 2 L or < 50% predicted*: Associated with increased postoperative pulmonary complications.
- *FEV_1 < 1 L*: Predicts poor secretion clearance, prolonged ventilation, difficult weaning, and possible need for tracheostomy [20].

3.3.8 Cardiac Imaging and Advanced Studies

- *Coronary angiography*: Should be reviewed preoperatively in MDT meetings for coronary anatomy, lesion location, degree of stenosis, and dominance [1].
- *CT aortography*: Indicated in patients with *dilated ascending aorta*, often associated with bicuspid aortic valve disease or aneurysmal dilation.
  - Findings guide surgical planning (e.g., simple tube graft replacement vs. *Bentall procedure*) with implications for anesthetic management.

- *CT chest*: Recommended for patients with prior *mediastinal radiation* or *redo sternotomy*, to evaluate sternal proximity to underlying cardiac structures.
- *Myocardial perfusion scanning (thallium/technetium)*: Differentiates *viable myocardium* (reversible perfusion defects) from *scar tissue* (irreversible defects).
- *Cardiac MRI*: Useful in differentiating partial vs. full-thickness infarctions, particularly in patients with poor ventricular function where the benefit of revascularization is uncertain.

3.3.9 Electrocardiography (ECG)

A baseline *12-lead electrocardiogram* should be obtained during the preanesthetic visit and compared with previous tracings to identify new ischemic changes or evolving cardiac pathology. Baseline rhythm should be documented, and abnormalities such as:

- *Atrial fibrillation*
- *Atrial flutter*
- *Heart block (any degree)*

must be clearly noted. Medication reconciliation should include review of ongoing *antiarrhythmic therapy* and rate/rhythm control drugs.

3.3.10 Echocardiography

Preoperative *echocardiographic evaluation* is of paramount importance and should be carefully reviewed at the *multidisciplinary team (MDT) meeting* prior to surgery, particularly in patients with valvular heart disease or those scheduled for ascending aortic surgery [1]. Key considerations include:

- Decision-making regarding *valve repair versus replacement*
- Detection of *coexisting valvular disease*
- Identification of *adult congenital anomalies* (e.g., patent foramen ovale [PFO], atrial septal defect [ASD]) that may require concomitant repair

If transthoracic echocardiography (TTE) is inconclusive, a *transesophageal echocardiogram (TEE)* may be requested for definitive assessment. Intraoperatively, TEE has become the *standard monitoring tool* for functional evaluation and guiding surgical decisions [17].

In patients with *coronary artery disease (CAD)*, particular attention should be paid to:

- *Regional wall motion abnormalities (RWMA)*
- Their correlation with the diseased coronary territories, which provides essential guidance for myocardial protection and revascularization planning [21] (Table 2).

Table 2 Echocardiographic findings and their impact on the anesthetic plan [22]

Structure	Findings of importance	Impact on anesthetic plan
Left ventricle (LV)	Ejection fraction (EF) Regional wall motion abnormalities (RWMA) LV thrombus or spontaneous echo contrast (SEC) LV diastolic function Dilated/ischemic cardiomyopathy	Monitoring with PAC or TEE Careful selection of induction agents Inotropic support if EF is low Consider mechanical circulatory support (MCS) prior to induction in severe cardiomyopathy Tailored IV fluid management
Right ventricle (RV)	RV systolic function RV filling status	RV inotropic support Tailored IV fluid management
Valvular lesions	Stenosis Regurgitation	Assessment of severity intraoperatively Plan for repair if lesion is > moderate
Aorta	Presence, site, and severity of atherosclerosis (especially ascending aorta)	Cautious aortic manipulation during cannulation and cross-clamping TEE-guided IABP placement Anticipation and early management of postoperative stroke risk
Pericardial disease/effusion	Tamponade physiology Constrictive pericarditis	Cautious induction with team preparedness Emergency readiness for pericardial drainage Anticipation of significant blood loss in constrictive pericarditis
Anatomical defects	Defect site, type, size, and shunt severity	Hemodynamic instability risk with severe shunts Potential volume overload
Intracardiac thrombus	Site and size of thrombus	Risk of systemic embolization

4 Risk Scores and Risk Stratification

Following comprehensive history taking, physical examination, and review of investigations, patients must be stratified according to established *risk scoring systems*. These scores estimate perioperative mortality and morbidity, guide clinical decision-making, and balance the *risk–benefit ratio* of cardiac surgery.

The most widely used system is the *European System for Cardiac Operative Risk Evaluation (EuroSCORE II)*, which has been validated internationally as a reliable predictor of operative mortality and as a benchmark for surgical quality assessment (Table 3) [24].

EuroSCORE II Risk Categories:

- *Low risk*: 0–3
- *Medium risk*: 4–7
- *High risk*: ≥8

Table 3 EuroSCORE II risk factors [23]

Category	Risk factors
Patient-related	Age, gender, chronic lung disease, extracardiac arteriopathy, poor mobility, previous cardiac surgery, active endocarditis, critical preoperative state, renal impairment, insulin-dependent diabetes
Cardiac-related	CCS Class IV angina, LV function (EF), recent myocardial infarction (within 90 days), pulmonary hypertension, NYHA class
Operation-related	Surgery on thoracic aorta, urgency of operation, procedural complexity ("weight of operation")

4.1 Definitions of Selected EuroSCORE II Variables

- *NYHA Class*:
  - I: No symptoms with moderate exertion
  - II: Symptoms with moderate exertion
  - III: Symptoms with mild exertion
  - IV: Symptoms at rest
- *CCS Class IV Angina*: Angina at rest or with minimal exertion.
- *Extracardiac arteriopathy*: Claudication, >50% carotid stenosis, prior amputation for vascular disease, or prior/planned intervention on abdominal aorta/limb arteries/carotids.
- *Renal dysfunction*:
  - Creatinine clearance 51–85 mL/min
  - Creatinine clearance ≤50 mL/min
  - On dialysis (any serum creatinine)
- *Critical preoperative state*: Includes VT/VF, aborted sudden death, CPR, mechanical ventilation, inotropic support, intra-aortic balloon pump or ventricular assist device preoperatively, or acute renal failure.
- *LV Function*:
  - Good: EF ≥ 51%
  - Moderate: EF 31–50%
  - Poor: EF 21–30%
  - Very poor: EF ≤ 20%
- *Urgency of procedure*:
  - Elective, Urgent, Emergency, Salvage (requiring CPR on way to OR).
- *Weight of procedure*:
  - Isolated CABG (baseline)
  - Single major non-CABG procedure (e.g., valve surgery, aortic replacement)
  - Two major procedures (e.g., CABG + valve replacement)
  - Three or more major procedures (e.g., CABG + AVR + MVR; Bentall procedure) (Tables 4, 5, and 6).

Table 4 ASA physical status classification

Class	Description
I	Normal healthy patient
II	Patient with mild systemic disease
III	Patient with severe systemic disease, not incapacitating
IV	Patient with severe systemic disease that is a constant threat to life
V	Moribund patient, not expected to survive 24 h with or without surgery

Table 5 Rockwood frailty index [25, 26]

Category	Description
Very fit	Robust, active, energetic, well-motivated
Well	No active disease, but less fit than "very fit"
Well controlled	Well-managed comorbid disease; symptoms stable
Apparently vulnerable	Slowed or symptomatic but not dependent
Mildly frail	Limited dependence in instrumental activities of daily living (IADLs)
Moderately frail	Requires assistance with IADLs and basic ADLs
Severely frail	Completely dependent in ADLs or terminally ill

Table 6 Code status categories [27]

Category	Resuscitative measures accepted
Full resuscitation	All measures: CPR, defibrillation, cardiac arrest medications, intubation and mechanical ventilation
Limited code	Selected measures only (e.g., CPR but no intubation/ventilation)
Do not attempt resuscitation (DNAR/DNR)	No resuscitation in cardiac/respiratory arrest; all other treatment continues
Comfort measures only	End-of-life care only; no resuscitation or aggressive interventions

5 Medication Reconciliation

5.1 Antiplatelet Agents

Medication reconciliation is a critical component of the preoperative assessment, particularly in patients scheduled for cardiac surgery, where perioperative hemostasis is often precarious. Special attention must be paid to *antiplatelet agents*, as these drugs are frequently prescribed in patients with ischemic heart disease, recent coronary stenting, or other cardiovascular comorbidities.

Table 7 Management of antiplatelet therapy before cardiac surgery [28, 29]

Drug	Recommendation
Aspirin (100–325 mg daily)	Continue preoperatively in CABG patients.
Clopidogrel/Ticagrelor	Discontinue ≥5 days before elective CABG. Discontinue ≥24 h before urgent CABG.
Prasugrel	Discontinue ≥7 days before elective CABG.
GP IIb/IIIa inhibitors (IV):	
Eptifibatide/Tirofiban	Discontinue 2–4 h before CABG.
Abciximab	Discontinue ≥12 h before CABG.

Failure to appropriately manage antiplatelet therapy may significantly increase the risk of:

- *Intraoperative surgical bleeding*
- *Reexploration for hemostasis*
- *Higher postoperative morbidity and mortality* [28, 29]

Therefore, a structured approach to reviewing, discontinuing, or bridging antiplatelet therapy is mandatory prior to surgery.

Table 7 summarizes the recommended guidelines for perioperative reconciliation of commonly used antiplatelet agents before cardiac surgery.

5.2 Anticoagulant Agents

Many patients presenting for cardiac surgery are on chronic anticoagulation due to conditions such as *atrial fibrillation, mechanical heart valves, or prior thromboembolic disease*. Perioperative management requires balancing the *risk of bleeding* with the *risk of thromboembolism.*

Bridging with *therapeutic low-molecular-weight heparin (LMWH)* may be required in selected high-risk patients, but unnecessary bridging increases perioperative bleeding risk (Table 8) [28, 29].

Table 8 Perioperative management of anticoagulants in cardiac surgery [28, 29]

Drug class/agent	Preoperative management	Bridging/reversal	Postoperative restart
Vitamin K antagonist (Warfarin)	Stop 3–5 days before surgery to normalize PT/INR.	Bridging with SC LMWH in high-risk patients. Emergency reversal: PCC (preferred) ± FFP; Vitamin K 5 mg IV/PO/SC (reduces INR in 12–24 h).	Resume 12–24 h after adequate hemostasis.
Direct thrombin inhibitor (Dabigatran)	Stop ≥48 h pre-op if normal renal function. Stop 2–4 days pre-op in severe renal impairment.	Bridging not required due to rapid onset/offset.	Resume when hemostasis secure.
Direct Factor Xa inhibitors (Rivaroxaban, Apixaban, Edoxaban)	Stop ≥48 h before surgery.	Bridging generally not required (consider in very high thromboembolic risk).	Resume when hemostasis secure.
Heparin bridging	Consider only in *very high-risk patients*: mechanical prosthetic valves, valvular AF (moderate-to-severe MS), AF with CHA_2DS_2-VASc >4, recent (<4 weeks) ischemic stroke, ACS, PE, LV apical thrombus, or antithrombin/protein C/S deficiency.	Use therapeutic LMWH (dose-adjusted).	Transition back to oral anticoagulation post-op.

PCC prothrombin complex concentrate, *CHA_2DS_2-VASc* clinical prediction rules for estimating the risk of stroke in people with nonrheumatic atrial fibrillation (AF)

5.3 Beta-Adrenergic Blockers

The majority of patients presenting for *coronary artery bypass grafting (CABG)* are prescribed *beta-adrenergic blockers* for the management of angina, hypertension, and atrial fibrillation. These agents confer several important perioperative benefits:

- *Reduction in 30-day mortality* following cardiac surgery [30, 31]
- *Myocardial protection*, including attenuation of ischemia–reperfusion injury
- *Control of perioperative arrhythmias*, particularly atrial fibrillation

Clinical Recommendation

Patients who are already established on beta-blocker therapy should *continue treatment throughout the perioperative period*, unless contraindicated by bradycardia, severe hypotension, or advanced heart block.

5.4 Angiotensin-Converting Enzyme Inhibitors (ACEIs) and Angiotensin II Receptor Blockers (ARBs)

The role of *ACE inhibitors (ACEIs)* and *angiotensin II receptor blockers (ARBs)* in the perioperative management of cardiac surgery patients remains a subject of debate.

- While these agents provide long-term benefits in the management of *hypertension, heart failure, and left ventricular dysfunction*,
- Their *perioperative use* in *CABG surgery* is associated with an increased risk of *intraoperative hypotension* and *vasoplegic syndrome*.

Clinical Recommendation

Given these concerns, many centers adopt the practice of *withholding ACEIs and ARBs in the immediate preoperative period* and resuming therapy postoperatively once hemodynamic stability is achieved [30, 31].

Statins

In patients with *coronary artery disease*, perioperative *statin therapy* provides significant protective benefits and is strongly recommended.

- *Continuation*: Patients established on statins should *continue therapy until surgery*.
- *Initiation*: If not previously prescribed, initiation is best deferred until after surgery, to avoid confounding perioperative adverse effects.
- *Benefits*: Established preoperative use of statins has been shown to:
  - Reduce the incidence of *postoperative atrial fibrillation (AF)*
  - Shorten *hospital length of stay*
  - Provide *pleiotropic vascular protection* beyond lipid-lowering effects [32]

Clinical Recommendation

Statin therapy should be *maintained perioperatively* in all cardiac surgical patients already receiving treatment.

5.5 Surgical Site Infection Prevention

Deep sternal wound infection (DSWI) remains a serious complication following cardiac surgery, and *Staphylococcus aureus carriage* in the skin and nasal passages has been identified as a major risk factor.

5.6 Preoperative Measures

- In *elective cardiac surgery patients* who are documented *S. aureus* carriers—or in those without confirmed negative screening—*intranasal mupirocin* (twice daily) is recommended, beginning *5 days prior to surgery*.

5.7 Intraoperative Antimicrobial Prophylaxis

- *Cefazolin* is the *first-line systemic antibiotic of choice*.
- In patients with a *penicillin allergy*, suitable alternatives include:
  - *Vancomycin*
  - *Clindamycin*
- In patients colonized with *methicillin-resistant Staphylococcus aureus (MRSA)*, *vancomycin* is the antibiotic of choice.

5.8 Atrial Fibrillation (AF) Prevention

Postoperative atrial fibrillation (POAF) is a common complication after cardiac surgery and is associated with increased morbidity, prolonged hospitalization, and higher healthcare costs. Several pharmacological strategies are available for its prevention.

5.8.1 Beta-Blockers

- *Continuation*: Patients already established on beta-blocker therapy should *continue treatment perioperatively*.
- *Initiation*: In patients not previously on beta-blockers, initiation *2–3 days prior to surgery* may reduce the incidence of POAF. Titration should be guided by *heart rate and blood pressure* tolerance.

5.8.2 Amiodarone

- *Efficacy*: A regimen of *6 days preoperatively followed by 6 days postoperatively* has been shown to be *more effective than beta-blockers* in reducing POAF incidence.
- *Limitations*: Its use is restricted by the higher rate of *acute toxicities* (e.g., bradycardia, hypotension) and *long-term complications* (e.g., thyroid dysfunction, pulmonary toxicity, hepatic effects).

5.9 Pain Prevention

Effective perioperative pain control is an essential component of enhanced recovery after cardiac surgery.

- *Analgesic adjuvants*: In selected patients, preoperative administration of *gabapentin* or *pregabalin* has been shown to reduce the severity of *postoperative pain* and improve analgesic outcomes.
- These agents may also contribute to *opioid-sparing effects*, reducing the need for high-dose narcotics and minimizing opioid-related side effects.

Clinical Consideration
Use should be individualized, taking into account patient comorbidities, renal function, and potential sedative effects.

6 Premedication

Premedication in cardiac surgical patients must balance the goals of anxiolysis, analgesia, and amnesia against the risk of he modynamic instability.

6.1 Night Before Surgery

- A *short-acting hypnotic*, such as *lorazepam 1–2 mg orally*, may be administered the night before s? > urgery to promote sleep [33].

6.2 Preoperative Holding Area / Induction Preparation

- A *short-acting intravenous benzodiazepine* (e.g., *midazolam 1–2 mg*) and/or a *short-acting opioid* (e.g., *fentanyl 50 mcg*) may be administered under anesthesiologist supervision, particularly during *intravascular catheter placement.*
- The use of benzodiazepines also helps reduce the risk of *implicit memory formation and awareness under anesthesia* [34].

6.3 Special Considerations

- *Careful dose titration* is essential in high-risk patients, such as those with:
  - *Critical aortic stenosis*
  - *Severe ventricular dysfunction*
  - *Extreme age (>80 years)* [35]

Clinical Recommendation: Premedication should be individualized, using the lowest effective dose to achieve anxiolysis and amnesia while minimizing hemodynamic compromise.

6.3.1 Admission to the Operating Theatre Suite

Upon arrival in the operating theatre, the patient is formally handed over to the anesthesia and surgical team, ensuring transfer of all pertinent clinical information.

Initial Assessment

- The anesthesiologist reassesses the patient's clinical status and determines the need for pre-induction *intravenous anxiolysis*.

Monitoring and Vascular Access

- *Standard monitors* (ECG, noninvasive blood pressure, pulse oximetry, capnography) are applied in accordance with ASA and cardiac anesthesia guidelines.
- A *wide-bore peripheral intravenous line* is established.
- A *radial arterial line* is inserted under local anesthesia for continuous invasive blood pressure monitoring and frequent arterial blood sampling.

Central Venous Access

- *Timing of insertion* depends on patient stability:
  - In *critically ill patients with poor cardiac reserve*, a *jugular central venous line* may be inserted *pre-induction* under local anesthesia, often with conscious sedation, to facilitate immediate vasoactive support.
  - In *stable patients*, central venous access is typically performed *after induction of anesthesia and tracheal intubation*, thereby reducing anxiety and discomfort.

Baseline Laboratory Assessment

- *Arterial blood gas (ABG)* and *activated clotting time (ACT)* are obtained before induction of anesthesia to guide intraoperative management.

6.3.2 Monitoring

Comprehensive intraoperative monitoring is essential in cardiac surgery to ensure patient safety, guide hemodynamic management, and detect complications at the earliest possible stage.

Standard Monitoring for General Anesthesia

- *Electrocardiography (ECG)*
- *Pulse oximetry*
- *Bispectral index (BIS)* for depth of anesthesia
- *End-tidal carbon dioxide ($ETCO_2$)*
- *Respiratory function monitoring* (tidal volume, airway pressure, minute ventilation)

Cardiac-Specific Standard Monitoring

- *Invasive arterial blood pressure monitoring* (typically radial artery; femoral line if severe peripheral vascular disease)
- *Central venous pressure (CVP)* monitoring

- *Nasopharyngeal temperature monitoring*
- *Intraoperative transesophageal echocardiography (TEE)*
  - TEE provides continuous, real-time assessment of ventricular function, valvular disease, and surgical repair.
  - Contraindications (absolute and relative) must be carefully assessed preoperatively [14].

Advanced Hemodynamic Monitoring

- *Central Venous Pressure (CVP)*: Historically considered the gold standard for preload assessment, but its reliability in predicting fluid responsiveness is limited, as it depends heavily on the Frank–Starling curve.
- *Alternative methods*:
  - *Pulmonary artery occlusion pressure (PAOP)* and *left ventricular end-diastolic dimension (LVEDD)* can provide more precise preload assessment, but are more invasive and require expertise.
  - *Dynamic indices* such as *pulse pressure variation (PPV)* and *stroke volume variation (SVV)* are increasingly used.
    - For example, a *pleth variability index (PVI) > 13%* is highly predictive of fluid responsiveness in mechanically ventilated patients in sinus rhythm [36].
  - These modalities are less invasive but require further validation in diverse patient populations.

Neuromonitoring

In select cases (e.g., *aortic dissection repair* or *complex valvular surgery*), *cerebral oximetry* using forehead sensors may be employed to assess regional cerebral oxygen saturation and reduce the risk of neurological complications [37].

6.3.3 Special Case: Type A Aortic Dissection

Definition and Urgency

Type A aortic dissection is defined as a *tear in the intimal layer* of the ascending aorta, allowing blood to track between the *media and adventitia*, creating a false lumen alongside the true lumen. This condition constitutes a *surgical emergency*, with mortality increasing by *1–2% for every hour of delay* between diagnosis and definitive surgical intervention [38, 39].

Life-threatening complications include:

- Cardiac tamponade
- Hemorrhagic shock
- Aortic rupture
- Acute aortic regurgitation
- Stroke
- Myocardial infarction

High-Risk Medical Conditions

- *Hypertension* (abrupt or transient severe elevations)
- *Genetically mediated aortic disease*
  - *Syndromic*: Marfan syndrome, Loeys–Dietz syndrome, vascular Ehlers–Danlos syndrome, Turner syndrome, familial aneurysm-osteoarthritis syndrome
  - *Nonsyndromic*: Familial aortic aneurysm/dissection, bicuspid aortic valve, aortic coarctation
- *Degenerative aortic disease*, including thoracic and abdominal aneurysms
- *Inflammatory disorders* (Takayasu arteritis, giant cell arteritis)
- *Aortic instrumentation, trauma, or surgery*

Clinical Presentation

- Severe, stabbing chest and/or back pain ("classic" feature)
- Echocardiographic evidence of an intimal flap in the ascending aorta
- New diastolic murmur (aortic regurgitation)
- Signs of malperfusion (stroke, limb ischemia, visceral ischemia)
- Hemodynamic instability [38, 39]

Diagnostic Evaluation

Gold standard: ECG-gated CT angiography of the entire aorta, which provides: [40]

- Location and extent of the intimal flap/dissection
- Sites of intimal tears and reentry points
- Involvement of cerebral vessels (guides cerebral protection strategies)
- Patency of femoral/axillary arteries (bypass cannulation options)
- Presence of thoracic or abdominal aneurysms
- Radiological evidence of malperfusion
- Pericardial/pleural effusion
- Degree of aortic calcification or intramural hematoma
- Anatomic anomalies (e.g., aberrant right subclavian artery, anomalous vertebral origins)

Echocardiography (TTE/TEE): Defines severity and mechanism of associated *aortic regurgitation* and detects pericardial tamponade [41].

Risk Assessment

Preoperative evaluation should document:

- Etiologic risk factors
- Comorbidities
- Signs of malperfusion (neurological deficit, abdominal pain, pulseless extremity) [42]

Poor prognostic indicators include:

- Age > 70 years
- Abrupt severe chest pain
- Hypotension, shock, or tamponade
- Renal failure at presentation
- Pulse deficit
- Abnormal ECG (especially ST elevation)
- Prior MI or AVR
- Visceral ischemia
- Severe pulmonary disease
- Syncope or stroke

Preoperative Preparation
- Baseline ECG, full laboratory panel, and cross-match (≥6 PRBC, 4 FFP, 2 platelets)
- *Emergency informed consent*
- ICU monitoring if awaiting OR readiness: bilateral radial arterial lines, central venous catheter under local anesthesia ± sedation
- *Aggressive blood pressure control*: short-acting IV beta-blockers (e.g., esmolol, labetalol) titrated to invasive BP monitoring, to reduce shear stress, limit aortic regurgitation, and minimize rupture risk [38]

Intraoperative Monitoring
- *Bilateral invasive arterial lines* to assess true vs. false lumen perfusion and arch involvement
- *Central and peripheral temperature monitoring* (for organ protection and hypothermic circulatory arrest if required)
- *Bispectral index (BIS)* and *bilateral cerebral oximetry* for brain monitoring during hypothermic arrest
- *Intraoperative TEE* for:
  - RWMA evaluation
  - Assessment of coronary ostial compression (commonly RCA) → may require bypass grafting
  - Confirmation of diagnosis in equivocal cases, particularly in extremis [43]

  Additional considerations:

- A *rapid infusion device* should be available at the start of surgery, given the risk of sudden exsanguination from aortic rupture.

6.3.4 Special Case: Acute Cardiac Tamponade

Definition
Cardiac tamponade is defined as the *accumulation of fluid under pressure within the pericardial sac*, leading to impaired ventricular filling, reduced cardiac output, and, if untreated, cardiovascular collapse and death. Tamponade may occur in an *acute* or *subacute* form [44].

Etiology

Causes include:

- Pericardial effusion of any origin (neoplastic, infectious, inflammatory, uremic)
- Hemopericardium due to trauma, aortic rupture, or myocardial rupture
- Iatrogenic causes (cardiac catheterization, pacemaker insertion, post-cardiotomy bleeding, percutaneous interventions)

Clinical Presentation

The clinical manifestations depend on both the *volume of fluid* and the *rate of accumulation*:

- *Acute tamponade*
  - Develops within minutes (e.g., trauma, cardiac/aortic rupture, procedural complications)
  - Presents as *cardiogenic shock* with chest pain, tachypnea, severe dyspnea
  - *Jugular venous distension* (often striking, with venous engorgement of forehead and scalp)
  - *Muffled heart sounds*
  - *Hypotension, tachycardia, and narrow pulse pressure* (Beck's triad)
  - Cool extremities, peripheral cyanosis, and oliguria due to low cardiac output
  - Pericardial fluid volume may be small because the *pericardium is noncompliant*
- *Subacute tamponade*
  - Develops over days to weeks (e.g., neoplastic, uremic, or idiopathic pericarditis)
  - Symptoms: progressive *dyspnea, chest fullness, peripheral edema, fatigue*
  - Signs: jugular venous distension, muffled heart sounds, and pulsus paradoxus

Additional Findings in Post-cardiotomy Tamponade

- *Arterial blood gases (ABG)*: metabolic lactic acidosis, reflecting tissue hypoperfusion
- *Laboratory findings*: anemia due to surgical or medical bleeding

Evaluation

In cardiac surgical patients—particularly *post-cardiotomy*—cardiac tamponade must be suspected in any patient presenting with *hemodynamic instability*.

- *Chest X-ray*: may demonstrate a *widened mediastinum* or an enlarged cardiac silhouette.
- *Bedside echocardiography*: the diagnostic tool of choice, confirming tamponade by detecting *pericardial fluid collection, right atrial/ventricular diastolic collapse*, and impaired ventricular filling [44, 45].

Preparation and Intraoperative Management

Once tamponade is *suspected or confirmed*, *emergency surgical intervention* or, in selected cases, *subxiphoid pericardiocentesis* must be initiated without delay.

Monitoring and Access

- In addition to standard intraoperative monitors, *invasive arterial blood pressure monitoring* is essential for beat-to-beat assessment.
- Establishment of *wide-bore intravenous access* is mandatory.
- If peripheral access is inadequate, a *central venous line* should be inserted pre-induction, allowing administration of *inotropic and vasopressor infusions* [46, 47].

Surgical Preparation

- The *surgical field must be scrubbed and draped prior to induction*, with the surgical team scrubbed and ready for an *emergency sternotomy or incision*, as patients are at risk of *sudden cardiovascular collapse during induction*.
- A *rapid fluid infuser* should be immediately available, particularly if tamponade is secondary to trauma or *aortic surgical leaks*, where sudden, massive hemorrhage may occur.

Anesthetic Considerations

1. *Induction technique* must be tailored to the patient's *hemodynamic status*.
2. The choice of induction agents should minimize *myocardial depression* and *hemodynamic instability*.
3. Preparedness for *immediate surgical decompression* is crucial, as circulatory collapse may occur at the moment of induction [46, 47].

6.3.5 Special Case: Mechanical Complications of Myocardial Infarction

Types of Mechanical Complications

Mechanical complications following acute myocardial infarction (MI) are rare but *catastrophic*, typically presenting as surgical emergencies with profound hemodynamic instability. These include:

1. *Acute severe mitral regurgitation* due to *papillary muscle rupture*
2. *Ventricular septal rupture (VSR)*
3. *Ventricular free wall rupture* [48]

Clinical Urgency and Evaluation

1. These complications usually occur in the setting of *acute MI with cardiogenic shock*, necessitating *emergency surgical intervention*.
2. *Diagnostic evaluation* should be expedited with *echocardiography* and/or *CT angiography*, both to confirm the diagnosis and to delineate the anatomical lesion.

3. In cases of *severe cardiogenic shock or impending cardiac arrest*, patients may require *mechanical circulatory support (MCS)* prior to surgery:
4. *Intra-aortic balloon pump (IABP)* counterpulsation
5. *Veno-arterial extracorporeal membrane oxygenation (VA-ECMO)*
6. *Impella device*
7. In extreme cases, *combined support (ECpella: Impella + VA-ECMO)* may serve as a bridge to surgery [49–51].

Timing of Surgery and MDT Role

1. The *Heart Team / MDT* must urgently determine optimal timing of intervention.
2. *Ventricular septal rupture (VSR)*: May be stabilized temporarily with inotropes and MCS to allow the necrotic septum to fibrose, improving chances of durable surgical repair.
3. *Ventricular free wall rupture*: Represents a *true surgical emergency*, often requiring immediate, sometimes *salvage surgery*.
4. *Papillary muscle rupture with severe mitral regurgitation*: Requires *emergent surgical repair or replacement*; medical therapy (afterload reduction with nitrates/nitroprusside, diuretics) may provide transient benefit if blood pressure permits, but many patients present in shock requiring inotropes, vasopressors, and IABP.

Anesthetic and Intraoperative Management

Pre-induction preparation:

1. Secure *wide-bore IV access*, invasive *radial arterial line*, and *central venous catheter*.
2. Infusions of *inotropes and vasopressors* should be connected, and in unstable patients, commenced *prior to induction*.
3. Consider pre-induction initiation of *MCS (IABP, VA-ECMO, Impella, or ECpella)* to stabilize circulation [49–51].

Intraoperative monitoring and support:

1. *Pulmonary artery catheter (Swan-Ganz)*: Introduced after induction; floated after cardiopulmonary bypass (CPB) initiation to monitor perioperative hemodynamics.
2. *Transesophageal echocardiography (TEE)*: Mandatory to:
3. Assess the lesion and severity
4. Guide surgical repair
5. Monitor real-time hemodynamics [14]
6. *Massive transfusion protocols* should be anticipated due to long, complex operations with *prolonged CPB and aortic cross-clamping*. A *rapid infuser system* must be available.

7 Conclusion

The *preoperative assessment* of patients undergoing cardiac surgery is a cornerstone of perioperative care. It allows not only for the *identification and optimization of comorbidities*, but also for the *stratification of surgical risk*, thereby guiding tailored anesthetic and surgical planning.

A thorough evaluation contributes to:

1. *Accurate risk estimation*, enabling prediction of morbidity and mortality and supporting strategies to minimize these risks.
2. *Optimization of medical conditions* prior to surgery, ensuring patients enter the operating room in the best possible state for favorable outcomes.
3. *Enhanced physician–patient rapport*, which facilitates cooperation, improves patient confidence, and contributes to reduced hospital length of stay.
4. *Patient and family education and counseling*, which remain essential components of care and should be consistently provided and documented.

In summary, preoperative evaluation represents both a *clinical and communicative process*, equally focused on improving outcomes and fostering trust between the patient, family, and multidisciplinary team.

References

1. Mihalj M, Carrel T, Urman RD, Stueber F, Luedi MM. Recommendations for preoperative assessment and shared decision-making in cardiac surgery. Curr Anesthesiol Rep. 2020;10:185–95.
2. Cornelissen H, Arrowsmith JE. Preoperative assessment for cardiac surgery. CEACCP. 2006;6(3):109–13.
3. Farasatkish R, Aghdaii NA, Azarfarin R, Yazdanian F. Can preoperative anesthesia consultation clinic help to reduce operating room cancellation rate of cardiac surgery on the day of surgery. Middle East J Anesthesiol. 2009;20(1):93–6.
4. Quinn TD, Wolczynski P, Sroka R, Urman RD. Creating a pathway for multidisciplinary shared decision-making to improve communication during preoperative assessment. Anesthesiol Clin. 2018;36(4):653–62.
5. Tylee MJ, Rubenfeld GD, Wijeysundera D, Sklar MC, Hussain S, Adhikari NK. Anesthesiologist to patient communication: a systematic review. JAMA Netw Open. 2020;3(11):e2023503.
6. Kaul P, Naylor CD, Armstrong PW, Mark DB, Theroux P, Dagenais GR. Assessment of activity status and survival according to the Canadian Cardiovascular Society angina classification. Can J Cardiol. 2009;25(7):e225–31.
7. Mahmoudi E, Kamdar N, Kim N, Gonzales G, Singh K, Waljee AK. Use of electronic medical records in development and validation of risk prediction models of hospital readmission: systematic review. BMJ. 2020;369
8. Mebazaa A, Pitsis AA, Rudiger A, Toller W, Longrois D, Ricksten SE, Bobek I, De Hert S, Wieselthaler G, Schirmer U, von Segesser LK. Clinical review: practical recommendations on the management of perioperative heart failure in cardiac surgery. Crit Care. 2010;14(2):1–4.
9. Rudiger A, Businger R, Streit M, Schmid ER, Maggiorini M, Follath F. Presentation and outcome of critically ill medical and cardiac-surgery patients with acute heart failure. Swiss Med Wkly. 2009;139(7–8):110–6.

10. Russell SD, Saval MA, Robbins JL, Ellestad MH, Gottlieb SS, Handberg EM, Zhou Y, Chandler B, HF-ACTION Investigators. New York Heart Association functional class predicts exercise parameters in the current era. Am Heart J. 2009;158(4):S24–30.
11. Schunk SJ, Zarbock A, Meersch M, Küllmar M, Kellum JA, Schmit D, Wagner M, Triem S, Wagenpfeil S, Gröne HJ, Schäfers HJ. Association between urinary dickkopf-3, acute kidney injury, and subsequent loss of kidney function in patients undergoing cardiac surgery: an observational cohort study. Lancet. 2019;394(10197):488–96.
12. Vives M, Hernandez A, Parramon F, Estanyol N, Pardina B, Muñoz A, Alvarez P, Hernandez C. Acute kidney injury after cardiac surgery: prevalence, impact and management challenges. Int J Nephrol Renov Dis. 2019:153–66.
13. Kara H. Preoperative carotid duplex scanning in patients undergoing coronary artery bypass grafting. Braz J Cardiovasc Surg. 2019;34:581–7.
14. Maus TM, Tainter CR, Herway ST. Introduction to basic perioperative and critical care echocardiography: examination, certification, indications, and contraindications. In: Essential echocardiography: a review of basic perioperative TEE and critical care echocardiography. Cham: Springer; 2022. p. 3–17.
15. Baran DA, Grines CL, Bailey S, Burkhoff D, Hall SA, Henry TD, Hollenberg SM, Kapur NK, O'Neill W, Ornato JP, Stelling K. SCAI clinical expert consensus statement on the classification of cardiogenic shock: this document was endorsed by the American College of Cardiology (ACC), the American Heart Association (AHA), the Society of Critical Care Medicine (SCCM), and the Society of Thoracic Surgeons (STS) in April 2019. Catheter Cardiovasc Interv. 2019;94(1):29–37.
16. Habib J, Baetz L, Satiani B. Assessment of collateral circulation to the hand prior to radial artery harvest. Vasc Med. 2012;17(5):352–61.
17. Prado-Olivares J, Chover-Sierra E. Preoperatory anxiety in patients undergoing cardiac surgery. Diseases. 2019;7(2):46.
18. Silvapulle E, Darvall J. Objective methods for preoperative assessment of functional capacity. BJA Educ. 2022;22(8):312–20.
19. Means Jr RT, Brodsky RA, Kunins L. Diagnostic approach to anemia in adults. UpToDate; 2022. Available at: https://www. uptodate. com/contents/diagnostic-approach-to-anemia-in-adults/print.
20. Adabag AS, Wassif HS, Rice K, Mithani S, Johnson D, Bonawitz-Conlin J, Ward HB, McFalls EO, Kuskowski MA, Kelly RF. Preoperative pulmonary function and mortality after cardiac surgery. Am Heart J. 2010;159(4):691–7.
21. Elsherbiny M, Abdelwahab Y, Nagy K, Mannaa A, Hassabelnaby Y. Role of intraoperative transesophageal echocardiography in cardiac surgery: an observational study. Open Access Maced J Med Sci. 2019;7(15):2480.
22. Ting PC, Wu VC, Liao CC, Chou AH, Tsai FC, Lin PJ, Chen CY, Chen SW. Preoperative right ventricular dysfunction indicates high vasoactive support needed after cardiac surgery. J Cardiothorac Vasc Anesth. 2019;33(3):686–93.
23. Nashef SA, Roques F, Sharples LD, Nilsson J, Smith C, Goldstone AR, Lockowandt U. Euroscore ii. Eur J Cardiothorac Surg. 2012;41(4):734–45.
24. Gao F, Shan L, Wang C, Meng X, Chen J, Han L, Zhang Y, Li Z. Predictive ability of European heart surgery risk assessment system II (EuroSCORE II) and the society of thoracic surgeons (STS) score for in-hospital and medium-term mortality of patients undergoing coronary artery bypass grafting. Int J General Med. 2021:8509–19.
25. Kovacs J, Moraru L, Antal K, Cioc A, Voidazan S, Szabo A. Are frailty scales better than anesthesia or surgical scales to determine risk in cardiac surgery? Korean J Anesthesiol. 2017;70(2):157–62.
26. Aguilar-Frasco JL, Rodríguez-Quintero JH, Moctezuma-Velázquez P, Morales-Maza J, Moctezuma-Velázquez C, Pastor-Sifuentes F, Medina-Franco H. Frailty index as a predictive preoperative tool in the elder population undergoing major abdominal surgery: a prospective analysis of clinical utility. Langenbeck's Arch Surg. 2021;406:1189–98.

27. Kaldjian LC, Erekson ZD, Haberle TH, et al. Code status discussions and goals of care among hospitalised adults. J Med Ethics. 2009;35(6):338–42.
28. Kreuziger LB, Karkouti K, Tweddell J, Massicotte MP. Antithrombotic therapy management of adult and pediatric cardiac surgery patients. J Thromb Haemost. 2018;16(11):2133–46.
29. Moster M, Bolliger D. Perioperative guidelines on antiplatelet and anticoagulant agents: 2022 update. Curr Anesthesiol Rep. 2022;12(2):286–96.
30. Wolf A, McGoldrick KE. Cardiovascular pharmacotherapeutic considerations in patients undergoing anesthesia. Cardiol Rev. 2011;19(1):12–6.
31. Mets B. To stop or not? Anesth Analg. 2015;120(6):1413–9.
32. Galyfos G, Sianou A, Filis K. Pleiotropic effects of statins in the perioperative setting. Ann Card Anaesth. 2017;20(Suppl 1):S43.
33. Bräuer A, Müller MM, Wetz AJ, Quintel M, Brandes IF. Influence of oral premedication and prewarming on core temperature of cardiac surgical patients: a prospective, randomized, controlled trial. BMC Anesthesiol. 2019;19:1–7.
34. Linassi F, Obert DP, Maran E, Tellaroli P, Kreuzer M, Sanders RD, Carron M. Implicit memory and anesthesia: a systematic review and meta-analysis. Life. 2021;11(8):850.
35. Rivasi G, Kenny RA, Ungar A, Romero-Ortuno R. Effects of benzodiazepines on orthostatic blood pressure in older people. Eur J Intern Med. 2020;72:73–8.
36. Scheeren TW, Ramsay MA. New developments in hemodynamic monitoring. J Cardiothorac Vasc Anesth. 2019;33:S67–72.
37. Vretzakis G, Georgopoulou S, Stamoulis K, Stamatiou G, Tsakiridis K, Zarogoulidis P, Katsikogianis N, Kougioumtzi I, Machairiotis N, Tsiouda T, Mpakas A. Cerebral oximetry in cardiac anesthesia. J Thorac Dis. 2014;6(Suppl 1):S60.
38. Malaisrie SC, Szeto WY, Halas M, Girardi LN, Coselli JS, Sundt TM, Chen EP, Fischbein MP, Gleason TG, Okita Y, Ouzounian M. 2021 The American Association for Thoracic Surgery expert consensus document: surgical treatment of acute type A aortic dissectionJ Thorac Cardiovasc Surg. 2021;162(3):735–58.
39. Gudbjartsson T, Ahlsson A, Geirsson A, Gunn J, Hjortdal V, Jeppsson A, Mennander A, Zindovic I, Olsson C. Acute type a aortic dissection–a review. Scand Cardiovasc J. 2020;54(1):1–3.
40. Budeanu RG, Broemmer C, Budeanu AR, Pop M. Comparing the diagnostic performance of ECG gated versus non-gated CT angiography in ascending aortic dissection: a GRRAS study. Tomography. 2022;8(5):2426–34.
41. Evangelista A, Maldonado G, Gruosso D, Gutiérrez L, Granato C, Villalva N, Galian L, González-Alujas T, Teixido G, Rodríguez-Palomares J. The current role of echocardiography in acute aortic syndrome. Echo Res Pract. 2019;6(2):R53–63.
42. Benedetto U, Dimagli A, Kaura A, Sinha S, Mariscalco G, Krasopoulos G, Moorjani N, Field M, Uday T, Kendal S, Cooper G. Determinants of outcomes following surgery for type A acute aortic dissection: the UK National Adult Cardiac Surgical Audit. Eur Heart J. 2022;43(1):44–52.
43. Jansen Klomp WW, Peelen LM, Brandon Bravo Bruinsma GJ, van't Hof AW, Grandjean JG, Nierich AP. Modified transesophageal echocardiography of the dissected thoracic aorta; a novel diagnostic approach. Cardiovasc Ultrasound. 2015;14(1):1–8.
44. Imazio M, De Ferrari GM. Cardiac tamponade: an educational review. Eur Heart J Acute Cardiovasc Care. 2021;10(1):102–9.
45. Kaemmerer AS, Alkhalaileh K, Suleiman MN, Kopp M, Hauer C, May MS, Uder M, Weyand M, Harig F. Pericardial tamponade, a diagnostic chameleon: from the historical perspectives to contemporary management. J Cardiothorac Surg. 2023;18(1):60.
46. Madhivathanan PR, Corredor C, Smith A. Perioperative implications of pericardial effusions and cardiac tamponade. BJA education. 2020;20(7):226.
47. Grocott HP, Gulati H, Srinathan S, Mackensen GB. Anesthesia and the patient with pericardial disease. Can J Anesth. 2011;58(10):952.
48. Damluji AA, Van Diepen S, Katz JN, Menon V, Tamis-Holland JE, Bakitas M, Cohen MG, Balsam LB, Chikwe J, American Heart Association Council on Clinical Cardiology, Council on Arteriosclerosis, Thrombosis and Vascular Biology, Council on Cardiovascular Surgery

and Anesthesia, Council on Cardiovascular and Stroke Nursing. Mechanical complications of acute myocardial infarction: a scientific statement from the American Heart Association. Circulation. 2021;144(2):e16–35.
49. Iida R, Kajiwara K, Saeki S, Ogawa S. Anesthesia for repair of ventricular septal rupture after acute myocardial infarction. J Clin Anesth. 2007;19(6):463–6.
50. Rob D, Špunda R, Lindner J, Rohn V, Kunstýř J, Balík M, Rulíšek J, Kopecký P, Lipš M, Šmíd O, Kovárník T. A rationale for early extracorporeal membrane oxygenation in patients with postinfarction ventricular septal rupture complicated by cardiogenic shock. Eur J Heart Fail. 2017;19:97–103.
51. Shibasaki I, Otani N, Saito S, Ogawa H, Masawa T, Tsuchiya G, Takei Y, Tezuka M, Kanazawa Y, Kanno Y, Yokoyama S. Overview of mechanical circulatory support for the management of post-myocardial infarction ventricular septal rupture. J Cardiol. 2022;

General Perioperative Care for Cardiac Surgery Patients

Amr Salah Omar and Sameh Ramadan Aboulnaga

EPICC module (lesson):	Cobatrice	
	Knowledge Note: please focus on specificities of the care of cardiac surgical patients (if any). EPICC team will then cross-reference to the general surgical care module where relevant.	Skills, attitudes and behaviours Note: please focus on specificities of the care of cardiac surgical patients (if any). EPICC team will then cross-reference to the general surgical care module where relevant.
General perioperative care of cardiac surgery patients (M. Wolff)	Perfusion management (overview) Management of patients following cardiac surgery (coronary grafting, valve replacement) and aortic surgery (arch, thoracic, abdominal) Surgical interventions in patients with acquired cardiac disease, perioperative management of the cardiovascular surgery patient and potential complications occurring within 24 h of cardiac surgery (note that detail on each major complications will be covered in a specific lesson), namely: Pain, sedation and delirium management Ventilation and weaning Coagulation and bleeding management Hemodynamic and fluid management Antibiotic prophylaxis Principles of minimal invasive surgery Indications for and methods of perioperative anti-thrombotic treatment Principles of cardiac pacing Management of endocarditis	Seek appropriate support and supervision in order to provide optimal patient care Assess conscious level and conduct a careful systems review Select & determine adequacy and route of administration of analgesia Document, monitor and manage fluid balance, circulating volume, drains, systemic oxygen supply Establish a plan for postoperative management

A. S. Omar (✉) · S. R. Aboulnaga
Department of Cardiothoracic Surgery/Cardiac Anesthesia & ICU Section, Heart Hospital, Hamad Medical Corporation, Doha, Qatar
e-mail: aelsid@hamad.qa

E. Elmistekawy, N. A. Shallik (eds.), *Perioperative Care of Cardiac Surgery Patients*, https://doi.org/10.1007/978-3-032-09817-7_3

1 Introduction

The existing burden of cardiovascular disease is significant in terms of mortality, morbidity and related costs. Cardiac surgery and related devices gain success in improving patient's survival.

The common existing cardiac surgeries include:

- Coronary artery bypass grafting
- Left ventricular aneurysm
- Ventricular septal rupture
- Heart valve repair or replacement
- Hypertrophic obstructive cardiomyopathy
- Aortic dissections
- Arrhythmia treatment
- Trans myocardial laser revascularization
- End-stage heart failure
  - Heart transplant
  - Surgery to place ventricular assist devices or total artificial hearts
- Pericardial disease
- Congenital heart disease atrial septal abnormalities
- Surgical approaches
  - *On-pump surgery*
  - *Off-pump heart surgery*

Cardiac surgeries place the patient in a critical situation that mandates collaborative work in order to prepare the patient for the next level of care [1, 2].

1.1 Learning Objectives

- After studying you should be able to
- Define principles of perfusion management
- Management of patients following cardiac surgery e.g. coronary grafting, valve replacement) and aortic surgery (arch, thoracic, abdominal)
- Surgical interventions in patients with acquired cardiac disease, perioperative management of the cardiovascular surgery patient and potential complications occurring within 24 h of cardiac surgery (note that details on each major complication will be covered in a specific lesson), namely:

  Pain, sedation and delirium management
  Ventilation and weaning
  Coagulation and bleeding management
  Hemodynamic and fluid management
  Antibiotic prophylaxis

- Principles of postoperative management of minimal invasive surgery
- Indications for and methods of perioperative anti-thrombotic treatment
- Principles of cardiac pacing
  Management of endocarditis

2 Management of Perfusion After Cardiac Surgery

2.1 Hemodynamic Management (Overview)

Perfusion management in cardiac surgery begins with comprehensive monitoring aimed at assessing cardiopulmonary function and facilitating the early detection of reversible conditions that may compromise myocardial performance or tissue perfusion.

2.2 Basic Perioperative Monitoring Includes

- Five-lead electrocardiogram (ECG) monitoring with ST segment analyses (Leads II, V)
- Noninvasive blood pressure measurement
- Invasive arterial blood pressure monitoring
- Pulse oximetry (SaO2 monitoring)
- End tidal carbon dioxide monitoring (ETCO2)
- Central venous pressure (CVP)

2.2.1 Central Venous Pressure (CVP)

- Measuring the CVP allows right ventricular filing assessment, and it is crucial for venous drainage monitoring on cardiopulmonary bypass (CPB)
- Central venous line insertion is usually done after anesthesia induction except in patients with hemodynamic compromise [2, 3].

2.3 Advanced Hemodynamic Monitoring

2.3.1 Swan-Ganz Catheterization

Swan-Ganz catheter remains one of the standards of hemodynamic monitoring for high-risk patients.

Cardiac output optimization could be achieved through early diagnosis and intervention of hypovolemia, which may prevent early onset of logistic multi-organ system dysfunction

Data that can be retrieved from the catheter include measurements of

- Continuous assessment of ventricular filling use central venous pressure
- (CVP) and pulmonary artery pressure (PAP)
- Pulmonary capillary wedge pressure (PCWP)

- Intermittent cardiac output (CO) determination
- Mixed venous gas sampling if indicated

Indications for Swan-Ganz catheters after cardiac surgeries include:

- Severe left ventricular dysfunction
- Poor distal vessels with poor revascularization hazards
- Severe hemodynamic instability
- Significant coexisting medical disease (pulmonary, cerebral, renal) [1, 2]

2.3.2 Transpulmonary Thermodilution and Calibrated Pulse Contour Analysis

Transpulmonary thermodilution and calibrated pulse contour analysis could substitute Swan-Ganz catheter for cardiac output monitoring after cardiac surgery. It is recommended to recalibrate these monitors regularly (4–8 h) and during extreme swifts in hemodynamics or after heart-lung machine weaning.

Precautions

- It may be inappropriate in patients with severe aortic insufficiency and those with peripheral vascular disease.
- It should not be used in patients with intra-aortic counter pulsation (IABC).
- Patients should be mechanically ventilated to be able to do continuous measurement of stroke volume variation (SVV) and pulse pressure variation (PPV)
- Cardiac arrhythmias limit the use of theses modalities

2.4 Perfusion

The postoperative course after cardiopulmonary bypass remains uneventful in many patients; but still it is poorly understood.

2.4.1 Physiological Variables

The physiological variables undergo extreme swings during this period including acid–base status, oxygen extraction, hemoglobin content, and carbon dioxide production.

Functional impairment characterizes cardio-circulatory dysfunction that follows cardiac surgeries. The reasons for this included hypertensive heart disease, congestive heart failure, different forms of cardiomyopathy, and microcirculatory disturbances.

2.4.2 Indicators of a Cardio-Circulatory Failure

- ScvO2 lactate more than 2.0 mmol/l
- Delayed capillary refill peripheral vasoconstriction (cold extremities corresponding to centralization).
- Arrhythmia [2, 3]

2.4.3 Goals for Cardio-Circulatory Therapy

The goal of fluid as well as positive inotropic and vasoactive drug management in postoperative cardiac surgery patients is sufficient to achieve tissue perfusion and a normalization of oxidative metabolism.

Cardiac output and O2 supply are dependent on adequate intravascular volume and cardiac function.

The recommended goals for postoperative cardiovascular therapy, as outlined by the Oxford Centre for Evidence-Based Medicine, serve as evidence-based targets for optimizing hemodynamic stability and organ perfusion following cardiac surgery.

- ScvO2 >70% or SvO2 >65%
- MAP (mean arterial pressure) >65 mmHg
- Cardiac Index >2.0 $l/min/m^2$
- CVP 8–12 mmHg (dependent on ventilation mode)
- LV-EDAI 6–9 cm^2/m^2
- ITBVI 850–1000 ml/m^2
- GEDVI 640–800 ml/m^2
- PAOP 12–15 mmHg
- Diuresis >0.5 ml/kgBW/h
- Lactate range less than 2.0 mmol/l [3, 4].

3 Management of Patients Following Cardiac Surgery (Coronary Grafting, Valve Replacement) and Aortic Surgery (Arch, Thoracic, Abdominal)

3.1 Basic Features of the Early Postoperative Period

1. Following cardiac surgeries, patients arrive in the ICU sedated and ventilated for several hours.

   Early extubation is referred to discontinuation of mechanical ventilation within 8 h of surgery. Proper analgesia is required with attempt to avoid respiratory depression.
2. Impairment of ventricular functions is common after cardiac surgeries on CPB as the heart suffers from ischemia and reperfusion effects. Additionally, diastolic dysfunction is common.
3. Adequate preload optimization is essential to obtain a better filing pressure through volume administration
4. Large fluid shift is expected. Urine output may be copious because of hemodilution during surgery. However, fluid administration is needed to keep intravascular volume optimized.
5. Surgery-related technical reasons and CPB-induced coagulopathy may cause mediastinal bleeding; therefore, chest drain monitoring is mandatory.
6. Hypothermia, which is referred to temperature (<36_C) on ICU admission, is associated with deleterious effects. Therefore, adequate rewarming should start late in surgery and actively completed in the ICU.

Hypothermia may predispose to atrial and ventricular arrhythmias, increase systemic vascular resistance, precipitate shivering, associated with platelet dysfunction and generalized coagulation defects, Increase the risk of wound infection [2, 3].

3.2 Management of Individual Cases

3.2.1 Coronary Artery Bypass Grafting (CABG)

3.2.1.1. Indications for surgery

Risk of adverse cardiac events is the main justification for CABG intervention

(a) Left main stem stenosis>50%
(b) Three-vessel disease with ejection fraction (EF) <50%
(c) Three-vessel disease with EF >50% and significant inducible ischemia on stress testing
(d) Two-vessel disease with involvement of proximal LAD and EF <50% or significant inducible ischemia on stress testing
(e) One- and two-vessel disease not involving the LAD with extensive myocardium in jeopardy but lesions not amenable to PCI

3.2.1.2. Preoperative considerations

1. Reduction of homogenous transfusion requirements could be achieved by preoperative autologous transfusion.
2. Anemia. Hematocrit <28% with acute coronary syndrome (ACS) is indication for preoperative transfusion. The risk of renal dysfunction, stoke and death could be increased with hemodilution during CPB to hematocrit <28%
3. Ischemia. Patients with critical stenosis should undergo aggressive treatment of potential ischemia through
   - Proper analgesia and sedation
   - Medications to control heart rate and blood pressure (intravenous nitrates and b-blockers),
   - Antiplatelet medications (aspirin, clopidogrel, heparin, IIb/IIIa inhibitors),
   - In refractory ischemia intra-aortic balloon pump (IABP) could be placed.
   - Heparin could be needed in ACS or with IABP, unfractionated heparin (UFH) could be continued up to the surgery time. However low-molecular-weight heparin (LMWH); but should be stopped 18–24 h before surgery [2, 3].
4. Medications management
   - Continuation of antianginal drugs in the morning of surgery including b-blocker
   - Aspirin could be continued up to the time of surgery and resumed after surgery when chest drainage is negative for 2 successive hours

- Clopidogrel should be stopped 5–7 days before elective surgery.
- Statins should be start or continued after surgery as it associated with reduced operative mortality, the risk of stroke, and the postoperative atrial fibrillation (POAF).

3.2.2 Off Pump Coronary Artery Bypass Grafting (OPCAB)

Indications: The adverse effects of CPB lead to implantation of OPCAB. Some evidences suggest that OPCAB is associated with less transfusion requirements, stroke, POAF, and AKI.

3.2.2.1. Conversion to on-pump cardiac surgery is occasionally required when

- Small, extensively diseased or intramyocardial coronary arteries.
- Poor LV function, cardiomegaly that make cardiac translocation difficult
- Development of arrhythmia or uncontrollable ischemia in spite of distal shunting.
- Intractable bleeding

3.2.2.2. Disadvantages

- The heart may not tolerate the manipulation required during off-pump surgery in severe LV dysfunction.

3.2.3 Minimally Invasive Direct Coronary Artery Bypass (MIDCAB)

Principle: Bypass the left anterior descending coronary artery (LAD) with graft from left internal mammary artery through small left anterior thoracotomy incision. The procedure could be combined with other vessels stenting in hybrid theatre.

3.2.4 Robotic or Totally Endoscopic Coronary Artery Bypass (TECAB)

Principle: It can be used to reduce the extent of the surgical incisions and reduce trauma to the patient through small ports. TECAB can be done with or without CPB, femoral cannulation if CPB is required [2, 3].

3.2.5 Valvular Surgeries

3.2.5.1. Aortic Stenosis (AS)
Indications for surgery

(a) Symptomatic AS (angina, dyspnea, syncope or post CPR)
(b) Asymptomatic AS (LV systolic dysfunction (EF <50%, abnormal response to exercise, extremely severe AS (AVA <0.6 cm^2, mean gradient >60 mm Hg) in severe AS or rapidly progressive valve

Preoperative considerations

1. Coronary angiography is indicated after 40 years age or in a younger patient with coronary risk factors, or a positive stress test.
2. Cardiac output may be severely affected in patients with AS when medications are given for ischemic symptoms preload, afterload, and heart

could be influenced by nitrate, calcium channel blockers, and B-blockers respectively.

3. Dental work should be instituted before surgery to reduce prosthetic valve endocarditis.
4. Patient age and contraindications to anticoagulation are key factors in determining the surgical approach, while the choice of valve type depends on these patient-specific considerations as well as clinical and anatomical factors.
5. Transcatheter aortic valve implantation (TAVI) involves the fluoroscopic-guided placement of a bioprosthetic valve via catheter in patients who are considered high-risk candidates for conventional open-heart surgery [2, 5, 6].

3.2.5.2. Aortic Regurgitation (AR)

Indications for surgery

Symptomatic patients with severe AR, Asymptomatic patients (EF <50%, severe LV dilatation, abnormal response to exercise).

Preoperative considerations

1. Vasodilators should be considered to reduce afterload, reduce regurgitation, and control hypertension.
2. B-blockers should be used with caution as it may increase regurgitation if bradycardia develops.
3. IABP is contraindicated.

3.2.5.3. Mitral Stenosis (MS)

Staging

>1.5 cm^2—"Progressive" –

1.1 to 1.5 cm^2—"Severe" –

1.2 ≤1.0 cm^2—"Very severe"

Indications for intervention

1. Percutaneous mitral balloon commissurotomy is recommended for symptomatic patients with severe MS (mitral valve area ≤1.5 cm^2, stage D) and favorable valve morphology in the absence of left atrial thrombus or moderate-to-severe MR (281–285, 287, 328). (Level of Evidence: A)
2. Mitral valve surgery (repair, commissurotomy, or valve replacement) is indicated in severely symptomatic patients (NYHA class III to IV) with severe MS (mitral valve area ≤ 1.5 cm^2, stage D) who are not high risk for surgery and who are not candidates for or who have failed previous percutaneous mitral balloon commissurotomy. (Level of Evidence: B) [2, 5, 6].

Types of intervention

1. Mitral valvuloplasty in patients with moderate or severe MS with acceptable echocardiography score (contraindicated in presence of LA thrombus, severe MR, severe TR or Wilkin score more than 8)

2. MV replacement
   - Symptomatic class I–II patients with severe MS and PA >60 mmHg (Class IIa) even if the patient is asymptomatic
   - Asymptomatic patients with MVA <1.5 cm^2 with recurrent embolism on anticoagulation if valve repair can be performed (Class IIb)

Preoperative considerations

- Atrial fibrillation worsens the hemodynamic performance (ventricular response needs control by b-blockers or calcium channel blockers, or continuing digoxin)
- Adequate preoperative diuresis to control edema
- Oral anticoagulation should be held 4 days before surgery, low-molecular-weight heparin (LMWH) could be considered if there is high risk of embolization to be stopped 18–24 h before proposed surgery [2, 5, 6].

3.2.5.4. Mitral Regurgitation (MR)

Mitral valve repair should be the preferred technique when it is expected to be durable (Class I).

Indication for surgery:

- Asymptomatic patients with LVEF >30% and end-systolic dimension <55 mm (Class I).
- Asymptomatic patients with LV end-systolic dimension ≥45 mm and/or LVEF ≤60% (Class I)

Surgery should be considered in the following situations in asymptomatic patients with:

- Preserved LV function and new onset atrial fibrillation or pulmonary hypertension (Class IIa)
- Preserved LV function and a high likelihood of durable repair, low surgical risk and flail leaflet, and LV end-systolic dimension ≥40 mm (Class IIa)
- Severe LV dysfunction refractory to medical therapy with a high likelihood of durable repair and low comorbidity (Class IIa)

Preoperative considerations

1. Acute mitral regurgitation (MR) is a medical emergency in which cardiac output is severely compromised. Supportive measures such as inotropes, vasodilators, and intra-aortic balloon pump (IABP) therapy can help stabilize the patient until definitive surgical or interventional therapy is undertaken.
2. Mechanical ventilation may be required for progressive hypoxia or hypercarbia.
3. Judicious use of diuretics in treating pulmonary edema
4. ACE inhibitors needed to improve forward flow.
5. Preload should be optimized to ensure forward output

3.2.5.5. Tricuspid Valve

Indications for surgery

- Tricuspid stenosis. Class III–IV HF symptoms, that are refractory to medical treatment
- Tricuspid regurgitation

(a) Class I: severe TR concomitant with MVD requiring surgery (TV repair).
(b) Class IIa: symptomatic severe primary TR.TV (repair or replacement)
(c) Class IIb: Less severe TR, annuloplasty is acceptable at the time of MV surgery
(d) Sepsis or recurrent pulmonary embolization from tricuspid valve vegetation.
(e) Class III: PA pressure <60 mm Hg and no mitral valve disease (considered) [2, 5, 6].

Preoperative considerations

1. Coagulation defects are expected due to elevation of pressures in the right side and passive liver congestion.
2. Hepatic function may be improved with diuretics and salt restriction but significant improvement in liver function tests may not be expected.
3. Adequate forward flow is obtained by having elevated central venous pressure [2, 5, 6].
4. A normal sinus rhythm provides better hemodynamics profile than with POAF [2].

3.2.5.6. Aortic Dissections

3.2.5.6.1. Pathophysiology

An aortic dissection occurs when false channel is created from a tear in the intima with blood passage to the media, which is contained by the adventitia and the outer layers. Progressive extension of the dissection with each cardiac contraction can lead to arterial wall weakening, rupture,
or branch vessel obstruction.

3.2.5.6.2. Classifications of Dissections

- Stanford type A (DeBakey type I–II, or proximal), dissection involves only the ascending aorta
- Stanford type B (DeBakey type III, or distal) aortic dissections involve the descending aorta without extension into the ascending aorta. Dissections are classified as acute when diagnosed within 14 days of symptom onset, and as chronic when identified beyond two weeks. (Fig. 1)

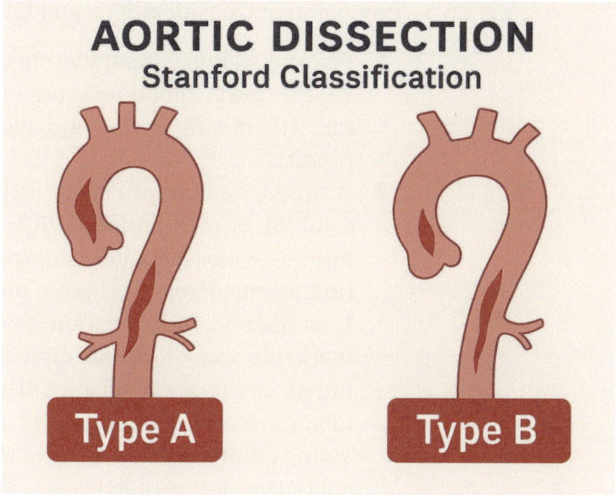

Fig. 1 Classification of aortic dissection. Type A dissections involve the ascending aorta. Type B dissections usually originate distal to the left subclavian artery and do not involve the ascending aorta. If they do extend retrograde, they are then considered type A dissections

3.2.5.6.3. Presentation

1. Type A dissection. This should be taken in consideration in differential diagnosis for patients presenting to the emergency department with acute chest pain. Missing the diagnosis could reach up to 40%. (The classical pain in AAD is tearing, ripping and radiating to the back, less common sharp pain that is non radiating could be encountered)
   - The possible complications include cardiac tamponade from hemopericardium, aortic regurgitation, stroke, and myocardial infarction.
   - Biomarkers, elevation in D-dimer could support the diagnosis suspicion
2. Type B dissection. This type is presented with back pain radiating to the abdomen. Possible rupture into the mediastinum, pleural spaces or abdomen could occur.

3.2.5.6.4. Indications for Surgery

1. Type A dissection. Surgery is indicated for all patients of acute and chronic type A dissection. The contraindications are relative patient age, development of renal, myocardial, or bowel infarction or massive stroke.
2. Type B dissections. Medical treatment is usually recommended for uncomplicated type B (surgical or endovascular procedures are offered for patients with complicated course e.g. hypertension, persistent pain, aneurysmal expansion or rupture, evidence compromise lower limbs)

3.2.5.6.5. Preoperative Considerations and Diagnostic Testing

1. Pharmacological treatment should be attempted upon suspicion to lower blood pressure (110 mm Hg SBP), the heart rate (to 60–70 bpm), and the force of cardiac ejection (dp/dt).
2. Antihypertensive of choice included a b-blocker (labetalol, esmolol, or metoprolol) with or without addition of sodium nitroprusside. Adequate control is essential until surgery time is mandatory in rupture prevention.
3. Examination of all extremities pulsations is essential to mark the extent of the dissection especially the carotid, radial, and femoral pulses. Differential blood pressure from upper to lower extremity is a clue to dissection diagnosis in young adult. Ejection systolic murmur over the aorta is also supportive to the diagnosis.
4. A comprehensive preoperative neurologic examination is mandatory (cerebral perfusion evidence is indication for emergency surgery).
5. Chest x-ray may show wide mediastinum or irregular aortic contour.
6. ECG is essential to exclude coronary origin of chest pain (nonspecific ST changes were noted in about 40% of patients and about 20% had ischemic insult)
7. CT scan with contrast should performed (90% sensitive and specific in identifying intimal flaps, evaluation of branches)
8. Transesophageal echocardiography is the procedure of choice for detecting intimal flaps, cardiac tamponade, and aortic regurgitation.
9. Transthoracic echocardiography may be to rule dissection in the ascending aorta, aortic regurgitation and to exclude pericardial effusion.
10. Magnetic resonance imaging (MRI) could be the most sensitive and specific but it is rarely required in emergency situations.
11. Coronary angiography is usually not required [2, 7].

3.2.5.7. Thoracic Aortic Aneurysms

3.2.5.7.1. Pathophysiology

Ascending aortic (AAo) aneurysms usually result from degeneration of the media or atherosclerosis.

3.2.5.7.2. Indications for Surgery

1. Ascending aortic aneurysms
   (a) Symptomatic, expanding, or more than 5.5 cm.

   (b) Aneurysms more than 5 cm associated with bicuspid aortic valves
   (c) Aneurysms more than 4.5 cm if there is surgery for aortic stenosis or regurgitation.
   (d) Aneurysms more than 4.5 cm in Marfan syndrome
   (e) Mycotic aneurysms
2. Transverse arch aneurysms
   (a) Ascending aortic aneurysms that require replacement that also extend into the arch.
   (b) Acute arch dissections with intimal tear in the arch or evidence of arch expansion or rupture
   (c) Aneurysms_5–6 cm in diameter
3. Descending thoracic (DAo) and thoracoabdominal aneurysms
   (a) Symptomatic aneurysms
   (b) Aneurysms_6.5 cm in diameter (atherosclerotic or chronic dissections)
   (c) Complicated acute type B dissections (uncomplicated if low risk patient)
4. Preoperative considerations
   1. Coronary angiography is required before surgery for ascending aortic and proximal arch aneurysms (not acute dissections)
   2. Myocardial perfusion stress imaging is indicated in patients with descending thoracic aneurysms because of the likelihood of coexistent CAD.
   3. A careful preoperative baseline neurologic evaluation is important because of the risks associated with circulatory arrest (stroke, seizures) and aortic cross-clamping (paraplegia).
   4. An assessment of aortoiliac disease is essential prior to any endovascular stenting procedure.
   5. Pulmonary status must be optimized prior to surgery.
   6. Renal function must be monitored carefully after angiography, especially in diabetic patients [2, 7].

4 Sedation, Analgesia, and Delirium Management

4.1 Fast Track Sedation (4–24 h Post-surgery)

4.1.1. All patients who undergo cardiac surgery should receive fast track sedation in the CTICU until they fulfil the criteria for extubation post cardiac surgery

4.1.2. Drugs for fast-track sedation
Propofol: Dose: 0.03–0.15 mg/kg (bolus)

5–50 mcg/kg/min (IV infusion via central line or a dedicated peripheral line)

4.1.3. Exceptions: Patients not deemed fit for fast tracking – Unstable hemodynamics, Significant bleeding.
Chest open
Advanced mechanical circulatory support through ECMO/LVAD

4.2 Short-term/intermediate Sedation (24–72 h Post-surgery or in the CCU)

4.2.1. All patients who don't fulfil criteria for fast track extubation, but who are expected to be weaned and extubated with 24–72 h post-surgery

4.2.2. Drugs for short term/intermediate sedation

Propofol—Dose: 0.03–0.15 mg/kg (bolus)
5–50 mcg/kg/min (IV infusion via central line or a dedicated peripheral line)
Midazolam: bolus—0.02-0.08 mg/kg and
Infusion—0.04-0.2 mg/kg/h (via central line or a dedicated peripheral line)

Dexmedetomidine: 0.2–1.5 mcg/kg/h (infusion via central line or a dedicated peripheral line)

4.3 Long-Term Sedation (>72 h)

4.3.1. All patients who are expected to be ventilated for more than 72 h

4.3.2. Daily assessment of need of continuing sedation needs to be done

4.3.3. Daily sedation vacation needs to be done.
Lorazepam: bolus—0.02–0.06 mg/kg
Infusion—0.01–0.1 mg/kg/h
Midazolam: bolus—0.02–0.08 mg/kg and
Infusion—0.04–0.2 mg/kg/h (via central line or a dedicated peripheral line)
Dose adjustments of the above-mentioned medications has to be made in accordance to existing pharmacy protocols in case of hepatic r and renal impairment [8–10].

4.4 Assessment of Sedation Depth

4.4.1 The Richmond Agitation-Sedation Scale

- RASS is used for measuring quality and depth of sedation in adult ICU patients
- Target: Richmond Agitation Sedation Scale (RASS): 0 to −3 (Table 1)

Table 1 Criteria to initiate weaning—short-term ventilation [18–22]

Criteria	Yes	No
Awake with stimulation- no agitation, acceptable pain control		
Adequate reversal of neuromuscular blockade as evidenced by sustained head lift and strong handgrip		
Core temperature >35.5 °C		
No focal neurological deficits, GCS >8		
No metabolic/electrolyte disturbance causing neurological/neuromuscular dysfunction		
Cardiac index >2.2 L/min/m^2		
Blood pressure stable at 100–120 systolic on low doses of inotropes (dopamine, & dobutamine ≤8 mcg/kg/min, adrenaline & noradrenaline ≤0.12 mcg/kg/min or equivalent), milrinone ≤0.5 mcg/kg/min, not on vasopressin		
Heart rate <120/min		
Absent life threatening arrhythmias		
No evidence of acute myocardial ischemia/graft dysfunction		
Absent major x ray abnormalities like marked pulmonary edema, pleural effusion, pneumothorax		
ABGs on full ventilation PaO_2/FIO_2 >150 $PaCO_2$ <50 mm Hg pH 7.30–7.50		
Absence of gross abdominal distension		
Excessive fluid overload ruled out		
Chest tube drainage <50 mL/h		
Hb above the transfusion trigger No major coagulopathy		

- Always ensure administration of optimal dosage of analgesia before initiating sedation
- Most uncomplicated patients in the ICU should be titrated to RASS score not less than −2. Rarely, a patient who is extremely ill may be targeted to a deeper sedation level of −3 or −4 if this will facilitate necessary care [11].

4.5 Daily Sedation Holds Guidelines

4.5.1 Defenition

1. Wean/stop sedation
2. Consider Decreasing Narcotics Infusion by 25–50%

4.5.2 Indications

Patients who are being mechanically ventilated and who are receiving a continuous sedation infusion for more than 24 h.

4.5.3 Contra-Indications

- Patients receiving neuromuscular blocking agents for any reason.
- Severe ARDS
- Patients requiring FiO2 ≥60%, or PEEP >10 cmH20 or, inverse inspiration/expiration ratio or prone ventilation
- Hemodynamically unstable patients—or Malignant Arrhythmias.
- Patients receiving compassionate care [11, 12].

4.5.4 Procedure for Sedation Holds

- The ideal level of sedation is to keep the patient comfortable and lightly asleep but easily aroused (RASS scale 0 to −3).
- The level of sedation should be monitored, chartered hourly, and the choice of drug, the dose and route of administration adjusted appropriately
- The need for daily sedation hold should be assessed by Critical Care Consultant on the morning ward round and documented on the daily review sheet
- If recommended by the Critical Care Consultant, the attending physician should perform the daily sedation hold at a convenient time in the morning, as described below:
  - Sedation infusion should be discontinued,
  - Consider decreasing narcotics infusion by 25–50%
  - Assess as part of sedation holds:
    - Pain
    - Delirium
    - When the patient is calm and can follow commands proceed to Spontaneous
    - Breathing Trial (SBT)
  - If patient becomes agitated (RASS score + 2 or above), no SBT, bolus should be given and the sedation infusion should be resumed.
  - If continued sedation is required, start at lower dose than given previously—50% of original or lowest effective dose during titration—the most recent titration dose (before reaching −1 RASS)
    - Administer a bolus and titrate gradually to reach the target sedation level as appropriate. Do not resume at the previous full rate to avoid oversedation.
    - Abort sedation holds if patient becomes unstable during procedure [12].

4.5.5 Assess for Spontaneous Breathing Trial (SBT)

4.5.5.1. Criteria for SBT

- Calm and cooperative
- Hemodynamically stable
- PEEP: <8
- FiO2: <60
- pH: >7.34
- SPO2: >90%

- Conduct SBT for 1 min:
  Mode: CPAP
  PEEP: 0
  Pressure Support Ventilation: 5–10 cm $H2O$
  $FiO2$: Unchanged
- After 1 min, calculate Rapid Shallow Breathing Index (RSBI):
  RSBI = Respiratory Rate/Tidal Volume in liters
  <105 = 80% success, continue to conduct SBT for up to 2 h
  >105 = 95% failure, return to previous ventilator settings

Conduct SBT for up to 2 h and continuously reassess if completes successfully, discuss plans for extubation after reviewing blood gases [13–15].

4.5.5.2. SBT Termination Criteria
Respiration Rate >35/min for >5 min
SpO2 <90% for >2 min
New Arrhythmias.
Heart Rate change 20% from baseline
Blood Pressure change 20% from baseline
Accessory muscle use
Increased anxiety/diaphoresis

Return patients who fail a SBT to their previous ventilator settings and re-screen in 24
Monitoring:
Continuous real-time monitoring of heart rate, blood pressure, and oxygen saturation is mandatory.

4.6 Analgesia

4.6.1 General Guidelines for Analgesia in ICU

- Evaluate the patient's sedation and pain together
- Conduct pain assessment using an appropriate pain scale
- Search for presence of pain
- Determine the time since the patient's last analgesic.
- Ensure consistent analgesic therapy.
- Start sedation therapy of agitated, critically ill patients only AFTER providing adequate analgesia and treating reversible physiological causes (e.g., hypoxemia, hypoglycemia, hypotension, and withdrawal from alcohol or other drugs).

4.6.2 Dose of Analgesic Medications

- Morphine: 0.1 mg/kg bolus +2–4 mg/h infusion.
- Fentanyl: 0.1–0.2 mcg/kg bolus +25–50 mcg/h infusion
- Remifentanyl: 0.1–0.15 μg/kg/min initially, then titrated in the range 0.006–0.74 μg/kg/min, depending on the levels of analgesia and sedation requirement.

4.6.3 Target: Non-verbal Pain Scale 0–2

Dose adjustments of the above mentioned medications has to be made in accordance to existing pharmacy protocols in case of hepatic and/or renal impairment

4.6.4 Titrating off Infusions:

The potential for opioid withdrawal should be considered for patients receiving high doses or 7 days of continuous therapy. Doses should be tapered systematically (i.e. 10–30%per day) to prevent withdrawal symptoms.

4.6.4.1. For break through analgesia, boluses can be repeated. If more than 2 boluses are required in an hour, consider increasing rate of infusion [8, 11, 15].

5 Weaning and Extubation After Cardiac Surgery

5.1 Purpose

To delineate an evidence-based protocol to guide weaning and extubation of mechanically ventilated patients in heart hospital

5.2 Definition

- **Weaning**—is the process of decreasing the amount of support that the patient receives from the mechanical ventilator, so the patient assumes a greater proportion of the ventilatory effort
- **Spontaneous breathing trial (SBT)**—patient spontaneously breathing through the endotracheal tube (ETT) for a set period of time (usually 30 min to 2 h) either without any ventilator support (eg, through a T-piece or with minimal ventilator support. Methods of minimal ventilator support for an SBT include a low level of PSV (e.g., 5–7 cm H_2O), automatic tube compensation (ATC), or continuous positive airway pressure (CPAP).
- **Rapid shallow breathing index (RSBI)**—ratio of respiratory frequency to tidal volume (f/VT)
- **P 0.1**—Airway occlusion pressure during initial 0.1 s of inspiration [16, 17].

5.3 Abbreviations

ABG	Arterial Blood Gas
BNP	brain natriuretic peptide
CICU	coronary intensive care unit
cmH$_2$O	centimetres of water
CPAP	continuous positive airway pressure
CPOT	critical care pain observation tool (CPOT)
CT-ICU	cardio-thoracic intensive care unit
ETCO2	end tidal carbon dioxide
FiO2	fraction of inspired oxygen concentration
GCS	Glasgow coma scale
Hb	hemoglobin
IABP	intra aortic balloon pump
LV	left ventricle
LVEF	left ventricular ejection fraction
mmHg	millimeters of mercury
PaCO2	arterial carbon dioxide tension
PaO2	arterial partial pressure of oxygen
PA	pulmonary artery
PCI	percutaneous coronary intervention
PEEP	positive end expiratory pressure
PS	pressure support
PSV	pressure support ventilation
SaO2	arterial oxygen saturation
SIMV	synchronized intermittent mandatory ventilation

5.4 Protocol for Weaning of Short-term Ventilated Patients <24 h

5.4.1 Assess Fitness for Early Weaning Upon Admission to the CT-ICU

Possible exclusion criteria for early weaning

5.4.2 Criteria for Weaning from Short-term Ventilation (Tables 1 and 2)

5.4.2.1. Central nervous system

- Awake with stimulation- No agitation, acceptable pain control—CPOT SCORE ≤ 2 (Table 3)
- Adequate reversal of neuromuscular blockade as evidenced by sustained head lift more than 5 s and strong handgrip
- Core temperature >35.5 °C
- No focal neurological deficits

Table 2 Extubation criteria in short-term ventilated patients [18–22]

Criteria	Yes	No
Patient awake without stimulation		
Maintained hemodynamic stability		
Acceptable respiratory mechanics Vital capacity >10–15 mL/kg Negative inspiratory force >25 cm H_2O Spontaneous respiratory rate <24/min Rapid shallow breathing index (respiratory rate/tidal volume in liters) <100 at PEEP ≤5 and pressure support ≤10 P 0.1 <4 cm water		
Acceptable ABGs on 5 cm or less of CPAP, PS 10 PaO_2/FIO_2 >150 PCO_2 <48 mmHg pH 7.32		

- No metabolic/electrolyte disturbance causing neurological/neuromuscular dysfunction

5.4.2.2. Hemodynamic Stability

- Cardiac index >2.2 L/min/m^2
- Blood pressure stable at systolic 100–140 on low doses of inotropes (dopamine & dobutamine ≤8 mcg/kg/min, adrenaline and noradrenaline ≤0.12 mcg/kg/min, milrinone ≤0.5 mcg/kg/min, no vasopressin)/off medications
- Heart rate <120/min
- No life-threatening arrhythmias
- No evidence of acute myocardial ischemia/graft dysfunction

5.4.2.3. Respiratory

- No major x ray abnormalities like marked pulmonary edema, pleural effusion, pneumothorax
- Satisfactory ABGs on full ventilation
  - PaO2/FIO2 >150
  - PaCO2 <50 mm Hg
  - pH 7.30–7.50

5.4.2.4. Gastrointesntinal

- No gross abdominal distension, nor rigidity or tenderness.

5.4.2.5. Hematological

- Chest tube drainage ≤50 mL/h
- Hb maintained above the transfusion trigger (7–10 g/dl) [2, 18, 19]

Table 3 The Critical-Care Pain Observation Tool (CPOT) [23]

Indicator	Score		Description
Facial expressions	Relaxed, neutral	0	No muscle tension observed
	Tense	1	Presence of frowning, brow lowering, orbit tightening and levator contraction or any other change (e.g. opening eyes or tearing during nociceptive procedures)
	Grimacing	2	All previous facial movements plus eyelid tightly closed (the patient may present with mouth open or biting the endotracheal tube)
Body movements	Absence of movements	0 or normal position	Does not move at all (doesn't necessarily mean absence of pain) or normal position (movements not aimed toward the pain site or not made for the purpose of protection)
	Protection	1	Slow, cautious movements, touching or rubbing the pain site, seeking attention through movements
	Restlessness/ agitation	2	Pulling tube, attempting to sit up, moving limbs/thrashing, not following commands, striking at staff, trying to climb out of bed
Compliance with the ventilator (intubated patient)	Tolerating ventilator or movement	0	Alarms not activated, easy ventilation
	Coughing but tolerating	1	Coughing, alarms may be activated but stop spontaneously
OR	Fighting ventilator	2	Asynchrony: blocking ventilation, alarms frequently activated
Vocalization (extubated patients)	Talking in normal tone or no sound	0	Talking in normal tone or no sound
	Sighing, moaning	1	Sighing, moaning
	Crying out, sobbing	2	Crying out, sobbing
Muscle tension	Relaxed	0	No resistance to passive movements

(continued)

Table 3 (continued)

Indicator	Score		Description
Evaluation by passive flexion and extension of upper limbs when patient is at rest or evaluation when patient is being turned	Tense, rigid	1	Resistance to passive movements
	Very tense or rigid	2	Strong resistance to passive movements or incapacity to complete them
Total	/8		

5.4.3 Weaning Process for Short-term Ventilation

5.4.3.1. Minimize sedation based on clinical judgment

5.4.3.2. Maintain the Fio2 at 0.5 or below with a PEEP of no more than 5–7.5 cmH 2O. If higher PEEP is used and oxygenation is satisfactory, lower the PEEP by 2.5 cm water decrements, over 10–15 min intervals to 5 cm H_2O before initiation of weaning.

5.4.3.3. Weaning is usually accomplished in the SIMV mode. The ventilator rate is reduced by two breaths every 30 min with observation of the Sao2, ETCO2.

Direct weaning to pressure support ventilation (PSV) may be acceptable if the patient is deemed to be capable of triggering effectively. PS level should be kept ≤10 cmH_2O. If the ABGs and respiratory mechanics are acceptable after a 30–60 min spontaneous breathing trial (SBT) on continuous positive airway pressure (CPAP) or pressure support ventilation, the endotracheal tube is removed.

Leak test if history of traumatic intubation

5.4.4 Signs of Weaning Failure

- Somnolence, agitation, or diaphoresis
- Systolic blood pressure increases by more than 20 mm Hg over baseline or to over 160 mm Hg
- Heart rate changes by more than 20% from baseline in either direction or to above 140/min
- Acute need for vasoactive medications
- Arrhythmias develop or become more frequent
- Respiratory rate increases more than 10 breaths/min or to over 35/min for 5 min
- PaO_2 falls >15% in comparison to the baseline before initiation of weaning or SaO_2 falls to less than 90%
- PCO_2 rises above 50 mmHg with respiratory acidosis (pH <7.30)
- Increase in pulmonary artery occlusion pressure >18 mmHg during SBT [19, 20].

5.4.5 Extubation Criteria

5.4.5.1. Patient is awake without stimulation

5.4.5.2. Acceptable respiratory mechanics

- Vital capacity >10–15 mL/kg
- Negative inspiratory force >25 cm H_2O
- Spontaneous respiratory rate <24/min
- Rapid shallow breathing index (respiratory rate/tidal volume in litres) <100
- P 0.1 <4 s

5.4.5.3. Acceptable ABGs on 5 cm or less of PEEP and 10 cm or less of pressure support

- PaO2/FIO2 >150
- PCO_2 <48 mm Hg
- pH 7.32–7.5

5.4.6 Post-extubation Considerations

- Consider NIV (noninvasive ventilation) for patients with
  - Compromised left ventricular function (LVEF <35%)
  - Obstructive sleep apnea
- Humidified oxygen
- Optimize analgesia
- Incentive spirometry & assistance with secretion drainage, early mobilization, VTE prophylaxis

5.4.7 Criteria for Weaning of Long Term (>24 h of Mechanical Ventilation) Ventilated and Coronary Intensive Care Unit Patients

5.4.7.1. Additional criteria to initiate weaning

- GCS >8. No major neurological ailments potentially interfering with airway protection
- ICU associated weakness ruled out based on clinical judgment
- Improve cardiac function (PCI if indicated, pacemaker for heart block)—Check for improvement of function as per echo/pro BNP, decreasing inotropic requirement
- Pleural effusions drained if significant
- Preserved spontaneous cough and secretions necessitating suction less frequent than 2 hourly.
- Sepsis ruled out/under control with antibiotics. No high grade pyrexia
- Nutritional status optimized—Albumin, phosphate

5.4.7.2. Weaning process for long-term ventilation

Weaning can be accomplished by gradual reduction of mandatory ventilator rate or by spontaneous breathing trial. Spontaneous breathing modes (pressure support ventilation/Continuous positive airway pressure) should be encouraged in all patients as much as tolerated. Typical minimally assisted spontaneous breathing trail should last 30 min-2 h (Tables 4 and 5).

Table 4 Criteria to initiate weaning—long-term ventilation

Criteria	Yes	No
Awake with stimulation- no agitation, acceptable pain control		
ICU associated weakness ruled out		
Core temperature >35.5 °C, <38		
GCS >8. No major neurological ailments potentially interfering with airway protection		
The active cardiac issues addressed (PCI, pacemaker), improving cardiac function as per echo/pro BNP, minimal/no inotrope requirement		
Pleural effusions drained if significant, chest infection controlled.		
Nutritional status optimized—Albumin, phosphate		
Sepsis ruled out/under control with antibiotics		

Table 5 Extubation criteria in long-term ventilated patients [18–22]

Criteria	Yes	No
Adequate mental status to protect the airway, preserved spontaneous cough and secretions necessitating suction less frequent than 2 hourly.		
Hemodynamic tolerance of the weaning process		
Acceptable respiratory mechanics Vital capacity >10–15 mL/kg Negative inspiratory force >25 cm H_2O Tidal volume 4-6 ml/kg Spontaneous respiratory rate <35/min Rapid shallow breathing index (respiratory rate/tidal volume in liters) <100 PEEP ≤5 and pressure support ≤10 P 0.1 less than 4 cm H_2O		
Acceptable ABGs on 5 cm H_2O or less of CPAP, 10 cm H_2O or less of PS Pao2 >70 mmHg on an FIO2 less than 0.5 Pco2 <48 mmHg pH 7.32		
Comfortable breathing pattern without diaphoresis, agitation or anxiety		
A cuff leak >110 mL with the cuff deflated		

5.4.7.3. Extubation criteria- in addition to (Table 2)

- Comfortable breathing pattern without diaphoresis, agitation, or anxiety;
- Respiratory rate <35/min
- Adequate mental status to protect the airway, initiate a cough, and raise
- Secretions
- Hemodynamic tolerance of the weaning process as delineated for short-term ventilated patients
- Respiratory mechanics and ABGs as in Sect. 5.4.2
- A cuff leak >110 mL with the cuff deflated [2, 18–22]

6 Management of Postoperative Bleeding

6.1 Purpose

To define and outline the management of coagulation and blood products usage in the setting of immediate postoperative cardiac surgery patients.

6.2 Abbreviations

ACT	activated clotting time
aPTT	activated partial thromboplastin time
DVT	deep venous thrombosis
ECG	electrocardiogram
FFPs	fresh frozen plasma
Hb	hemoglobin
Hct	hematocrit
INR	international normalized ratio
NA	not applicable
PC	platelet concentrate
PRBCs	packed red blood cells
PT	prothrombin time
PvO2	central venous oxygen tension
rFVIIa	recombinant activated factor VII
SvO2	central venous oxygen saturation
TEG	thromboelastogram

6.3 All Post-cardiothoracic Surgical Patients Should Be Carefully Monitored for

- Vital signs, urine output recorded as per unit protocol
- Hourly chest tube drainage output
- Coagulations studies: platelet count, PT, aPTT, INR, ACT, fibrinogen level and TEG/ROTEM
- Hemoglobin level should be closely monitored hourly basis through ABG or VBG.
- Signs of cardiac tamponade (see appendix) should be regularly monitored and thought about
- TEG/ROTEM at second hour if the bleeding at first 2 h $\geq$100 ml/h

6.4 Maintain Hemodynamic, Temperature, and Metabolic Status,

- Systolic blood pressure 90–120 mmHg, mean arterial pressure ≥60 mmHg
- Temperature 36–37.5 °C
- Treat acidosis
- Manage shivering if present

6.5 Maintain Intravascular Volume and Oxygen Delivery, Transfuse PRBCs or Give Intravenous Fluids According to the Hemoglobin Levels For a Hemoglobin Level <7 g/dL: Transfuse PRBCs to Maintain Hb Levels Between 7 and 10 g/dL

6.5.1. **For a hemoglobin level between 7 and 9.9 g/dL consider PRBCs transfusion if any of these are present:**

- Patient's age more than 65 years
- Preoperative poor cardiac function (EF <35%)
- SvO_2 <65% or PvO_2 <30 mmHg
- History of cerebrovascular accidents in the past.
- Persistent chest tube drainage of more than 100 mL/h for 2 consecutive hours at any point.

6.5.2. **For a hemoglobin level ≥10 g/dL give intravenous fluids to maintain an adequate intravascular volume**

6.6 Correct Coagulation Abnormalities

6.6.1. **Give 25–50 mg protamine if bleeding continues with an ACT ≥150 s**

6.6.2. **Transfuse a pool of platelets if:**

- There is presence of active bleeding with a platelet count <50,000 per mL or,
- Abnormal platelet function is evidenced by TEG/platelet mapping with active bleeding regardless of the number of platelets or,
- When the platelet count is <20,000 per mL regardless of the bleeding volume

6.6.3. **Transfuse FFPs or Prothrombin complex concentrate:**

- Elevated aPTT, or INR (≥1.5) with continuous bleeding or,
- Clotting factor deficiency evidenced by TEG or,
- Massive transfusion (≥1 estimated total blood volume within 24 h)

6.6.4. **Give fibrinogen concentrates if:**

- Fibrinogen level is less than 1 g/L with continuous chest tube drainage
- Fibrinolysis evidenced by TEG

6.6.4.1. Fibrinogen dosage:

- If fibrinogen level is unknown: give 70 mg/kg
- If fibrinogen level known
  - Dose given (mg/kg) = target fibrinogen—present fibrinogen blood levels (mg/dL)/1.7

6.6.5. **Transfuse cryoprecipitate if:**

- Fibrinogen level <1 g/L (with no other indication for FFP transfusion)
- TEG evidence of dysfibrinoginemia
- Uremic bleeding, patients with chronic renal failure that have a blood loss

6.6.5.1. Cryoprecipitate dosage: 1 unit for every 7–10 kg patient's weight

6.6.6. **Give tranexamic acid if:**

- Patient received clopidogrel until less than 7 days prior to surgery
- Unexplained bleeding with normal platelet count
- Bleeding after prolonged cardiopulmonary bypass, >180 min
- TEG evidence of fibrinolysis
- Redo surgery

6.6.6.1. Tranexamic acid dosage:

- 15 mg/kg intravenous bolus followed by 1 mg/kg/h intravenous infusion or
- 20–30 mg/kg intravenous bolus as a single dose

6.6.7. **Give 1 g calcium chloride if:**

- Low ionized calcium level in laboratory blood test –Keep around 1
- Blood products transfusion in patients with hepatic impairment based on ionized calcium level (check on a half hourly basis if multiple transfusions are given)
- Rapid transfusion (≥10 units/h) even in patients with normal hepatic function

6.6.8. **Give desmopressin if:**

- Bleeding uremic patient
- Known case of Von-Willebrand disease

6.6.8.1. Desmopressin dosage: 0.3–0.4 mcg/kg intravenous bolus (in 50 mL of saline over 15–30 min)

6.6.9. **Timing of antiplatelets and DVT prophylaxis**

- Start aspirin not before the sixth postoperative hour and the drainage from the chest tubes is less than 50 mL/h for two consecutive hours unless otherwise advised by the surgical team
- Clopidogrel in the first postoperative day after removal of the chest tube, if indicated- Not earlier than 24 h after skin closure .
- Start DVT prophylaxis according to protocol in the first postoperative day if not contraindicated

6.7 Surgical Re-exploration Is Indicated If: Consider Rearrangement or Earlier in the Document (Lifesaving)

6.7.1 Excessive Chest Tube Output

- 500 ml during the first hour
- 400 ml during each of the first 2 h
- 300 ml during each of the first 3 h
- 1000 ml in total during the first 4 h
- 1200 ml in total during the first 5 h
- Sudden increase in drainage (>300 ml/h which has been minimal before)

6.7.2 Clinical Evidence of Cardiac Tamponade

- Low cardiac output state (oliguria, metabolic acidosis and prolonged rewarming)
- Raised airway pressure
- Raised central venous pressure
- Radiologic or echocardiographic signs of tamponade
- Unexplained tachycardia

6.8 If All Previous Measures Fail to Control the Bleeding Consider rFVIIa in a Bolus of 35–70 mcg/kg (After Discussion with ICU and Surgery Consultants)

- Caution, FFPs and platelets should be transfused prior to rFVIIa to give substrate to this medication to work

6.9 Interpretation and Management of TEG Abnormalities

6.9.1 Normal Values

- **R** (reaction time to initiate fibrin formation) = 3.7–8.3 min
- **K** (time and kinetics for fibrin cross-linkage) = 0.5–3.7 min
- **α Angle**(speed of clot strengthening): 46.8–73.6 degrees

- **MA** (maximum amplitude- fibrin and platelet interaction/aggregation) = 54.5–72.5 mm
- **LY30** (measured fibrinolysis 30 min after MA) = 0–7.5%
- **CI** (coagulation index- linear combination of R, K, MA, and α) = −3–3

6.9.2 Treatment Protocol for TEG Abnormalities

6.9.2.1. R time prolongation

- Between 14 and 21 min: 1 unit FFP
- Between 21 and 28min: 2 units FFP
- ≥28 min: 4 units FFP

6.9.2.2. MA

- <48 mm: 1 pool Platelet Concentrate
- <40 mm: 2 pools Platelet Concentrate

6.9.2.3. LY30

- LY30 at 7.5% or greater, with CI (coagulation index) less than 1.0: Tranexamic acid
- LY30 at 7.5% or greater, with CI greater than 3.0: patient is in hypercoagulability state, anticoagulate

6.9.2.4. R less than 3 min MA greater than 75 mm G greater than 15 K: patient is in hypercoagulability state, anticoagulante [24].

6.9.3 Platelet Mapping

- Performed in patients who were on aspirin, Clopidogrel or GP IIb/IIIa antagonists.
- Special kits are available for both aspirin as well as Clopidogrel, GP IIb/IIIa antagonists

6.9.3.1. Important notes:

- Always treat when the numbers correlate clinically (the patient is actively bleeding)
- Always rule out heparin as a cause of R prolongation (use heparinase)

6.9.3.2. Known Risk of Perioperative Bleeding Include

- Urgent/emergency procedure
- Redo operation, aortic surgeries

- Last dose of Clopidorel less than 5 days, Recent use of heparin and derivatives
- Hepatic/renal dysfunction
- Bleeding disorders
- Prolonged cardiopulmonary bypass >180 min [25–33].

7 Arrhythmia Prevention

7.1 Background

Postoperative atrial fibrillation (POAF) remains a major risk after cardiac surgery. About 12% of patients admitted to this unit postcardiac surgery experienced POAF, which led to hemodynamic instability, increased risk of stroke, and increased length of postoperative intensive care unit stay.

7.2 Definitions

1. Post cardiac surgery AF is defined as a new onset of AF after surgery during hospitalization.
2. Persistent AF: episodes last more than 7 days and may require either pharmacologic or electrical intervention to terminate.
3. Permanent AF: persisted for more than 1 year, either because cardioversion either failed or not been attempted.
4. Paroxysmal AF: episodes that terminated spontaneously within 7 days (most episodes last less than 24 h)
5. Controlled AF: exertional heart rate verified to be less than 110 beats/min and more than beats/min.
6. Transient AF: non-persistent episode, in theabsence of history of paroxysmal or persistent AF.

7.3 Patient Group

7.3.1. Patients with newly developed AF after surgery with or without hemodynamic instability.

7.3.2. Patients with persistent or permanent AF associated with or without rapid ventricular response (ventricular rate >100/min).

7.4 Prophylaxis Agaisnt Postoperative AF (Fig. 2)

7.4.1. *Pharmacologic*: In patients undergoing cardiothoracic surgery the risk of postoperative AF should be reduced by the administration of one of the following (Table 6):

7.4.1.1. Beta-blockers, re-institution of B-blockers for prophylaxis within 24 h of surgery.

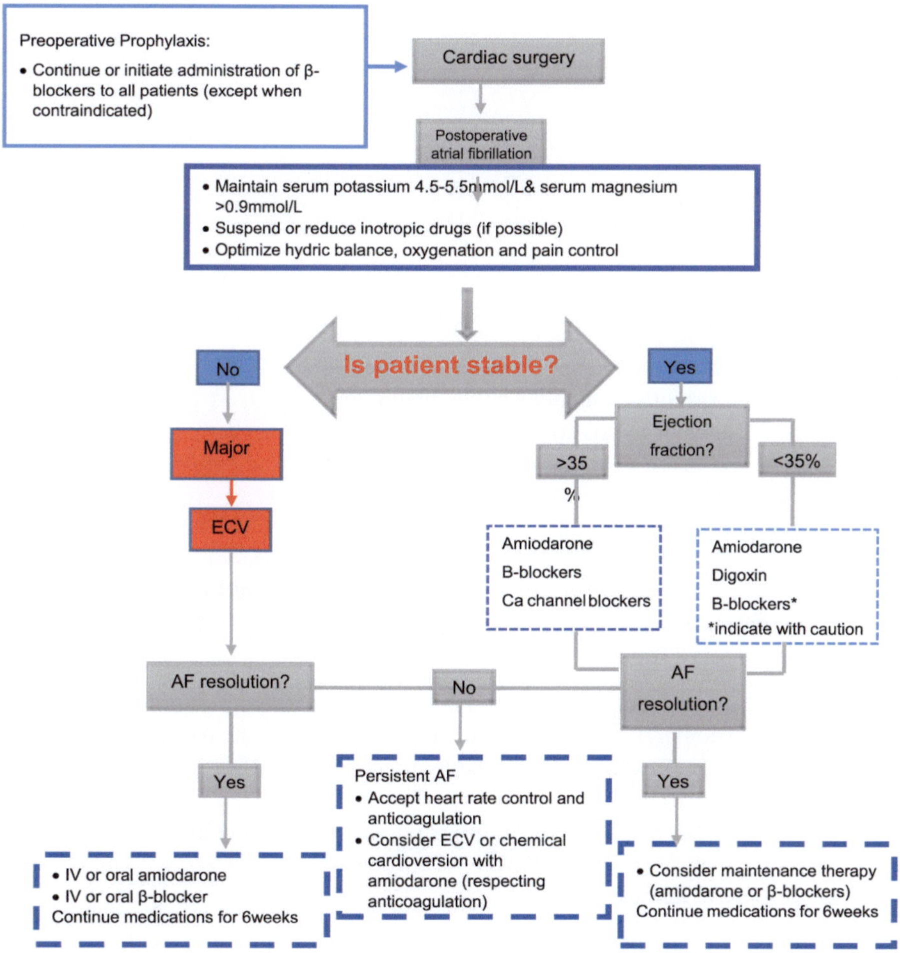

Fig. 2 Management of Postoperative AF [36]

Table 6 Summary of clinical recommendations for pharmacologic prophylaxis in postoperative AF

Drug	Strength of recommendation
Beta-blockers	A
Sotalol	B
Amiodarone	B
Verpamil	D
Diltiazem	D
Magnesium	D
Digoxin	I
Digoxin and prporanolol	C
Dexamthazone	I
GIK	D
Insulin	D
Triiodothyronin	D
Procianmide	D
Alinidine	D
Quinidine	D

GIK glucose insulin potassium

7.4.2. *During prophylaxis*

7.4.2.1. Appropriate use of antithrombotic therapy in AF patients, and
7.4.2.2. Correction of identifiable precipitants (such as electrolyte imbalance or hypoxia).

7.5 Treatment Options

7.5.1. *Rhythm-control strategy* unless contraindicated, should be the initial management option for the treatment of postoperative AF following cardiothoracic surgery (Table 4).

7.5.1.1. Amiodarone is recommended for patients with depressed left ventricular function who do not need urgent electrical cardioversion (hemodynamically unstable, under sedation).
7.5.1.2. Electrical cardioversion (Sect. 8.2)
7.5.1.3. Sotalol and class 1A antiarrhythmic drugs (procinamide and disop) may be used in patient with coronary artery disease without congestive heart failure.

7.5.2. Unless contraindicated, postoperative AF following non-cardiac surgery should be managed as for *acute-onset AF with any other precipitant* (Fig. 2 and Table 7)

7.5.3. *Pharmacologic ventricular response rate control*

7.5.3.1. Use B-blockers in patients who do not require urgent cardiovesion.
7.5.3.2. Non-diihydropyridine calcium channel blockers are recommended as second line agents [34–37]

Table 7 Summary of clinical recommendations for cardiac pacing to prevent postoperative AF

Intervention	Strength of recommendation
Right atrial pacing	I
Left atrial pacing	I
Biatrial pacing	B

Table 8 Clinical recommendations of pharmacologic rhythm control of postoperative AF

Drug	Strength of recommendation
Amiodarone[a,b]	E/C
Sotalol[b]	C
Class IA	C
Ibutilide	C
Beta-blockers	I
Calcium channel blockers	I
Digoxin	I
Class IC	D
Dofetilide	D

[a]Recommended agent for individuals with depressed left ventricular function or heart failure
[b]Recommended agent for patients with coronary artery disease but no heart failure

Table 9 Summary of clinical recommendations for pharmacologic rate control of postoperative AF

Drug	Strength of recommendation
Beta-blockers	B
Calcium channel blockers	B
Amiodarone[a,b]	I
Digoxin	I
Propafenon	D
Dofetilide	D

[a]Recommended agent for individuals with depressed left ventricular function or heart failure
[b]Recommended agent for patients with coronary artery disease but no heart failure

Digoxin and agents with proarrhythmic effects as dofetilide or agents with relative contraindication in CHD as flecainide and propafenone, have little efficacy (Tables 7, 8, and 9).

7.6 Prevention of Thromboembolism and Anticoagulation Role

7.6.1 Patients on Long-term Anticoagulant

Stop therapy at least 3 days before surgery, restart oral anticoagulant therapy after surgery, as soon as risk of bleeding is minimal. Bridge heparin therapy for patients at high risk of an embolic complication while off oral anticoagulant.

Table 10 CHADS-VASC score, thromboembolic risk, and effect of warfarin anticoagulation [38, 39]

Clinical parameter	Points
Congestive heart failure (any history)	1
Hypertension (prior history)	1
Age ≥75 years	1
Diabetes mellitus	1
Stroke, transient ischemic attack, or thrombembolism	2
Vascular disease	1
Age 65–74	1
Female	1

CHADS-VASC score of 0. Patients are considered to be at low risk with a score of 0, at intermediate risk with a score of 1 or 2, and at high risk with a score ≥3

7.6.2 Patients Not Ttaking Anticoagulant Prior to Cardiac Surgery

Thromboembolic risk increases significantly in patients with atrial fibrillation (AF) lasting more than 48 hours, particularly among those with high-risk features such as rheumatic mitral valve disease, prior thromboembolism, hypertension, or heart failure. These patients should be anticoagulated promptly to reduce the risk of systemic embolism and stroke. (Tables 8 and 10)

8 Management and Principles of Cardiac Pacing

8.1 Temporary Epicardial Pacemaker Leads Are Implanted During Cardiac Surgery on the Epicardial Surface of the Heart to Help in Rate and Rhythm Management Postoperatively

Pacing is required in only 25% and 10% in those undergoing valve and CABG procedures respectively

8.1.1. **Components**: any pacing system included electrodes and a generator; the former is in contact with the heart while the later strike electrical impulses.
8.1.2. **Epicardial Leads and Lead Systems**: Two electrodes are required to generate an electrical signal: a negative pacing electrode (anode) must remain in direct contact with the atrium and/or ventricle to deliver current to the myocardium, while a positive or grounding electrode (cathode) returns the signal to the generator to complete the electrical circuit.
8.1.3. **Settings**: The used epicardial wires and the patient demands determine the optimal pacing code.

A 3-letter code system used to describe the chamber(s) paced, chamber(s) sensed, and mode of operation, whereby A = atrial, V = ventricular, D = dual, O = none, and I = inhibited.

8.1.4. Pacing Modes Are either

(a) Synchronous as AAI, VVI, and DDD as the device senses intrinsic cardiac activities and the respond by competitive pacing inhibition.
(b) Asynchronous ventricular and dual pacing modes (i.e., DOO and VOO) are not recommended, as the sensing property is lacking with arrhythmia hazard from the "R-on-T" phenomenon (used only in the operating theatre when electrical interference from cautery devices exists)
(c) In general, cardiac output is improved with increasing the pacing rate within range. VVI pacing maintain the HR but without an atrial activity.
(d) The default sitting for stimulation (Output) is 10 mA, with maximum limits of 20 (A) and 25 (V) mA (this is used to control the amount of electricity). High energy tend to exhaust the battery life with minimal or no danger to the heart
(e) Sensitivity settings set the amplitude needed for intrinsic ECG complex recognition, in millivolts (mV). Sensing needs an impulse with adequate amplitude to pass the sensing threshold.
(f) Time delay is measured between the atrial signal onset (P wave) and subsequent ventricular activity (QRS), the A-V delay adjusted automatically on HR basis. Prolonging this parameter can be quite useful in fostering intrinsic ventricular activity in patients needing rate stimulation, thus promoting more physiological cardiac contraction versus right ventricular (RV) paced beats, while encouraging return of native conduction. In cardiac surgery patients with impaired ejection fraction.
(g) Cardiac output may increase from 10% to 20% with biventricular pacing in comparison to right ventricular pacing.
(h) Atrial pacing during surgery has advantages of diagnosing and treating atrial arrhythmias. Overdrive pacing particularly could terminate atrial flutter and some supraventricular tachycardia.
(i) Removal is typically done through gentle traction, the electrode usually dislodges from the heart and then withdrawn from the chest wall completely. Alternatively, they can be pulled in flush with the skin, cleansed, and clipped, retaining a portion of the wire inside the chest.

8.1.5. Troubleshooting

(a) Continuous increases in milliamperes to maintain pacing should be considered at risk for loss of capture and use of alternate pacing systems explored. Acute loss of capture mandates increasing the milliamperes, securing all connections, or suppressing the "EMERGENCY" button on certain devices
(b) Failure to sense, indicated by a pacing spike in or near a complex without indication for pacing, can be life-threatening as in R-on-T.
(c) Complications of temporary epicardial pacing included chamber perforation, infection, tamponade, and vascular injury.

8.1.6. Temporary transvenous pacemaker leads: under general anaesthesia or sedation with local Anesthesia subclavian vein cannulation under fluoroscopy to ensure appropriate lead placement, directed towards right ventricular apex. Perioperative antibiotics should be given.

8.1.7. Indications for pacing

Symptomatic patients with

- High degree AV block (third, Mobitz type I, or Mobitz type II)
- Sinus node dysfunction
- Sino-atrial block
- Sinus bradycardia
- Atrial pacing in AV dys-synchrony (especially in heart failure patients) [40–42].

9 Antibiotic Prophylaxis

- Postoperative infections may follow a fulminant or subacute clinical course.
- Virtually all patients have fever, tachycardia, chest pain or sternal instability, or purulent discharge.
- Bacteraemia is common occurring in 57% of patients with postoperative mediastinitis

9.1 Data from Several Studies Support the Prophylactic Antibiotic

- A single preoperative dose is as effective as a 5-day course
- Should target the anticipated or expected organisms in the facility.
- Complicated, contaminated, or dirty procedures should receive additional post-operative coverage
- During prolonged procedures, re-administered every 4 h (with exception of aminoglycosides, vancomycin and fluroquinolones).
- Administered within 1 h prior to incision.
- In cases of delayed skin closure (open chest), Routine antibiotic prophylaxis is cephazoline 50 mg/kg at the induction of anesthesia and on the bypass, then switching to vancomycin and imipenem

9.2 Empiric Antimicrobial Is Indicated

- When the likelihood of infection is high.
- Evidence of severe sepsis or severe organ dysfunction
- When the patient is immunocompromised (e.g. neutropenia) [43–45].

10 Principles of Minimally Invasive Cardiac Surgery

10.1 Background: Minimally Invasive Cardiac Surgery Is Based on Smaller Incision and Included

- Minimally invasive direct coronary artery bypass (MIDCAB): The principle is to bypass the left anterior descending coronary artery (LAD) with graft from left internal mammary artery through small left anterior thoracotomy incision. The procedure could be combined with other vessels stenting in hybrid theatre.
- Robotic or totally endoscopic coronary artery bypass (TECAB): The principle is to reduce the extent of the surgical incisions and reduce trauma to the patient through small ports. TECAB can be done with or without CPB, femoral cannulation if CPB is required.

10.2 Advantages

- Reducing the wound infection risks,
- Avoid the complications related to sternum healing,
- Reduced post-operative atrial fibrillation,
- Rreduced length of ICU and hospital stay,
- Early mobilization, and
- Better cost-effectiveness compared to traditional cardiac surgery.

10.3 Complications

- Left minithoracotomy may be associated with increase in operation time,
- Involvement of the intercostal nerves may be associated with more pain, and
- Increases length of mechanical ventilation time in some reports

10.4 Outcome(s)

- Associated with significantly longer aortic cross-clamp time
- Associated with longer CPB times
- Longer total surgery time
- Shorter length of ICU and hospital stay but longer ventilation time
- No difference in the incidence of perioperative myocardial infarction,
- No difference in the incidence of neurologic complications or stroke [46].

11 Endocarditis Management

11.1 Background

- Infective endocarditis (IE) is a lethal disease if untreated. It accounts for up to 1% of all severe hospital sepsis
- It is endovascular microbial infection of cardiovascular structures occur in sites of damaged endothelium caused by foreign bodies or turbulent flow.
- 41,000 hospitalized cases of IE reported annually
- One month mortality is about 30%
- CHF is developed in 33% of patients with IE
- In-hospital mortality (without CHF) is 13%

11.2 Pathogenesis

- Endothelial damage predisposes to platelets and fibrin deposition on the endothelial surface, with generation of non-bacterial thrombotic endocarditis (NBTE), when this associated with bacteremia leads to generation of infective vegetation.

11.3 Susceptible Patients

- Acquired valvular heart disease with stenosis or regurgitation
- Prosthetic heart valve
- Structural congenital heart disease, including surgically corrected or palliated structural
- Conditions, but excluding isolated atrial septal defect, fully repaired ventricular septal
- Defect or fully repaired patent ductus arteriosus, and closure devices that are judged to be deendothelialized
- Previous infective endocarditis
- Hypertrophic cardiomyopathy
- Non-cardiac factors
  - Precondition for bacterial adhesion, e.g., hepatic cirrhosis, leukemia
  - Impaired immune function
  - Compromised local non-immune defense mechanisms e.g. AV fistulae for hemodialysis
  - Broken skin (e.g. bed sores), or ICU (lines), hemodialysis patients or intravenous drug abusers all increase chances of having bacteremia.

11.4 Antibiotic Prophylaxis Recommendations

- Prosthetic heart valves or prosthetic material
- Valve repair
- History of endocarditis
- Heart transplant with abnormal valve function
- Certain congenital heart defects
- Cyanotic heart disease, not fully repaired
- Within 6 months of repair of defect
- Repairs with residual defects and/or leaks

11.5 Diagnosis

- The most important factor for the diagnosis of endocarditis is a high index of suspicion
- At least 2 sets of blood cultures
- Modified Duke Criteria for suspected IE
- Transthoracic recommended in those with suspected IE
- Assess for vegetations
- Assess hemodynamic severity of valve lesions
- Assess cardiac function
- Re-evaluation for clinical change/symptoms

11.6 Modified Duke Criteria

- Definite infective endocarditis
- Clinical Criteria 2 Major criteria, or1 Major criterion and 3 minor criteria, or • 5 Minor criteria
- Major criteria
  - Blood culture positive
  - Typical microorganism for IE (multiple variations)
  - Endocarditis by imaging study
  - Causative organisms (Streptococci, Viridians streptococci, Enterococci, Other streptococci, Staphylococci, Coagulase-negative, Coagulase-positive, Gram-negative organisms, Fungi, and HACEK organisms)

11.7 Echocardiography Criteria

- Evidence of endocarditis
  - Oscillating intracardiac mass on valve or supporting structures, in the path of regurgitant jets, or on implanted material in the absence of an alternative anatomic explanation, or
  - Abscess, or
  - New partial dehiscence of prosthetic valve, or
  - New valvular regurgitation
- Transthoracic resolution can detect 3–4 mm vegetation, sensitivity: 62–82%, specificity: 91–100% and readily available, usual approach to start with.
- Transesophageal resolution detects 1–2 mm vegetation, sensitivity: 87–100%, specificity: 91–100%, higher sensitivity in prosthetic valves

11.8 Treatment

11.8.1 Medical

- In uncomplicated cases treatment should be started only when the results, including antibiotic sensitivities, of the initial blood cultures are obtained. This may require re-culturing and waiting up to 8 days in a patient who has recently received antibiotics.
- In cases complicated by active sepsis, severe valvular dysfunction, conduction defects or infective emboli, empirical bactericidal antibiotic therapy should be started after three blood cultures have been taken.
- Laboratory
  - Baseline full blood count and measurement of renal and liver function should be obtained and repeated with a surveillance blood culture obtained at 72 h.
  - C-reactive protein (CRP) should be measured at the start of therapy and then daily
- Persistent fever beyond the first week of therapy often indicates the development of a complication

11.8.2 Surgical

Early cardiac surgical input regarding indications for operation is essential in:

- Valve dysfunction/ADHF
- Resistant organisms: Staph Aureus, Fungus
- Heart block or abscess formation
- Large mobile vegetation
- Persistent positive blood cultures
- Prosthetic valve endocarditis
- Recurrent embolization [47–50].

12 Postoperative Considerations Following Commonly Performed Procedures

12.1 Atrial Fibrillation (AF)

12.1.1. Background: Postoperative atrial fibrillation (POAF) is one of the major adverse events after cardiac surgery. The incidence of POAF is 30% for coronary artery bypass surgery and 40% for valvular surgeries.

The reason is usually predisposition, withdrawal of b-blockers and poor atrial preservation during surgery.

12.1.2. Consequences included thromboembolism, hemodynamic compromise, increase length of ICU stay and mortality.

12.1.3. Preventive strategies

- Early initiation of b-blockers
- Magnesium sulfate has been shown in some studies to reduce the incidence of POAF
- Amiodarone prophylaxis in patients at higher risk.
- Rate control could be an alternative in case of rhythm control failure [2, 51].

12.2 Postoperative Ischemia/Infarction

12.2.1. Background: Ischemia and infarction are frequent after cardiac surgeries; diagnosis of a perioperative myocardial infarction (PMI) can be difficult. Carful interpretation of the postoperative ECG should be done.

12.2.2. Causes of post-operative ischemia included inadequate myocardial protection, poor revascularization or impaired myocardial perfusion due to acute graft occlusion, coronary spasm or anastomotic stenosis

12.2.3. Management

- intravenous nitroglycerin
- Calcium channel blockers
- Echocardiography
- Insertion of IABP
- Angiography followed by percutaneous coronary intervention or reexplanation may be indicated if ST elevation noted in multiple leads

12.3 Perioperative Myocardial Infarction (PMI)

12.3.1. Background: The PMI could follow coronary artery surgery 4% (whether on- or off-pump) or isolated valvular surgeries as well 2%. The PMI correlate with adverse outcomes

12.3.2. Contributors to increased cardiac enzymes included recent myocardial infarction (AMI) before the surgery, perioperative myocardial infarction (PMI), poor cardiac protection, reperfusion related injury, and surgical trauma. Non coronary related enzyme rising occur in acute pericarditis, acute heart failure (AHF), renal failure, sepsis or rhabdomyolysis.

12.3.3. Diagnosis: The universal PMI diagnosis require increase in the CK-MB by more than 5–10 times the 99th percentile upper reference level plus either new pathological Q-waves or left bundle branch block (LBBB) on 12 lead electrocardiogram (ECG), image evidence of loss of viable myocardium, or angiographic evidence of new native or graft occlusion [2, 52, 53].

12.4 Acute Kidney Injury

12.4.1. Background: Acute kidney injury (AKI) complicates recovery from cardiac surgery in up to 30% of patients.

12.4.2. Diagnosis: The consensus definition proposed by the Acute Kidney Injury Network. Here, AKI was defined as an abrupt (within 48 h) reduction in kidney function, with absolute increase in the serum creatinine concentration of 0.3 mg/dL or greater (26.4 μmol/L) or a percentage increase of 50% or greater (1.5-fold from baseline).

12.4.3. Preventive strategies: Renal perfusion maintenance and adequate intravascular volume while avoiding venous congestion, administration of balanced salt fluid as opposed to high-chloride, and limitation of cardiopulmonary bypass time [54–56].

References

1. Griffiths MJ, Cordingley J, Price S. Cardiovascular critical care. Wiley; 2011.
2. Bojar RM. Manual of perioperative care in adult cardiac surgery. Wiley; 2011.
3. Jakob SM, Ruokonen E, Takala J. Assessment of the adequacy of systemic and regional perfusion after cardiac surgery. Br J Anaesth. 2000;84(5):571–7.
4. Carl M, Alms A, Braun J, Dongas A, Erb J, Goetz A, Goepfert M, Gogarten W, Grosse J, Heller AR, Heringlake M. S3 guidelines for intensive care in cardiac surgery patients: hemodynamic monitoring and cardiocirculary system. Ger Med Sci. 2010;8:12.
5. Vahanian A, Alfieri O, Andreotti F, Antunes MJ, Barón-Esquivias G, Baumgartner H, Borger MA, Carrel TP, De Bonis M, Evangelista A, Falk V. Guidelines on the management of valvular heart disease (version 2012). Eur Heart J. 2012;33(19):2451–96.
6. Nishimura RA, Otto CM, Bonow RO, Carabello BA, Erwin JP, Guyton RA, O'Gara PT, Ruiz CE, Skubas NJ, Sorajja P, Sundt TM. 2014 AHA/ACC guideline for the management of patients with valvular heart disease. Circulation. 2014:CIR-0000000000000031.
7. Hagan PG, Nienaber CA, Isselbacher EM, et al. The international registry of acute aortic dissection (IRAD). New insights into an old disease. JAMA. 2000;283:897–903.
8. Patel SB, Kress JP. Sedation and analgesia in the mechanically ventilated patient. Am J Respir Crit Care Med. 2012;185(5):486–97.
9. ICU Sedation-Guidelines of care; San Diego Patient Safety Council, December 2009.

10. Shapiro MB, West MA, Nathens AB, Harbrecht BG, Moore FA, Bankey PE, Freeman B, Johnson JL, McKinley BA, Minei JP, Moore EE, Maier RV. Inflammation and the host response to injury large scale collaborative research project. J Trauma. 2007;63:945–50.
11. Ely EW, Truman B, Shintani A, Thomason JWW, Wheller AP, Gordon S, et al. Monitoring sedation status over time in ICU patients: the reliability and validity of the Richmond Agitation Sedation Scale (RASS). JAMA. 2003;289:2983–91.
12. Kress JP, Pohlman AS, O'Connor MF, Hall JB. Daily interruption of sedative infusions in critically ill patients undergoing mechanical ventilation. N Engl J Med. 2000;342:1471–7.
13. Sessler CN, Gosnell MS, Grap MJ, Brophy GM, O'Neal PV, KeaneKA, Tesoro EP, Elswick RK. The Richmond Agitation–Sedation Scale: validity and reliability in adult intensive care unit patients. Am J Respir Crit Care Med. 2002;166:1338–44.
14. Adult critical care guidelines for sedation and analgesia in the intubated patient-Critical Care Directorate Nottingham University Hospitals NHS Trust.
15. Stone P, Phillips C, Spruyt O, Waight C. A comparison of the use of sedatives in a hospital support team and in a hospice. Palliat Med. 1997;11:140–4.
16. Jeganathan N, Kaplan CA, Balk RA. Ventilator liberation for high-risk-for-failure patients: improving value of the spontaneous breathing trial. Respir Care. 2015;60(2):290–6.
17. Dres M, Teboul J-L, Monnet X. Weaning the cardiac patient from mechanical ventilation. Curr Opin Crit Care. 2014;20(5):493–8.
18. Kaplan JA, Reich DL, Konstadt SN. Kaplan's cardiac anesthesia: expert consult premium. Elsevier Health Sciences; 2011.
19. Marino PL. Marino's the ICU book. Lippincott Williams & Wilkins; 2013.
20. Haas CF, Loik PS. Ventilator discontinuation protocols. Respir Care. 2012;57(10):1649–62.
21. Klein A, Vuylsteke A, Nashef SAM. Core topics in cardiothoracic critical care. Cambridge University Press; 2008.
22. Coplin WM, Pierson DJ, Cooley KD, Newell DW, Rubenfeld GD. Implications of extubation delay in brain-injured patients meeting standard weaning criteria. Am J Respir Crit Care Med. 2000;161(5):1530–6.
23. Gélinas C, Fillion L, Puntillo KA, Viens C, Fortier M. Validation of the critical-care pain observation tool in adult patients. Am J Crit Care. 2006;15(4):420–7.
24. Maul TM, Massicotte MP, Wearden PD. ECMO biocompatibility: surface coatings, anticoagulation, and coagulation monitoring. In: Extracorporeal membrane oxygenation-advances in therapy, vol. 3; 2016. p. 27–61.
25. Klein AA, Arnold P, Bingham RM, Brohi K, Clark R, Collis R, Gill R, McSporran W, Moor P, Rao Baikady R, Richards T, Shinde S, Stanworth S, Walsh TS. AAGBI guidelines: the use of blood components and their alternatives 2016. Anaesthesia. 2016;71(7):829–42. https://doi.org/10.1111/anae.13489. Epub 2016 Apr 8
26. American Society of Anesthesiologists Task Force on Perioperative Blood Management. Practice guidelines for perioperative blood management: an updated report by the American Society of Anesthesiologists Task Force on Perioperative Blood Management. Anesthesiology. 2015;122(2):241–75. https://doi.org/10.1097/ALN.0000000000000463.
27. Kozek-Langenecker SA, Afshari A, Albaladejo P, Santullano CA, De Robertis E, Filipescu DC, Fries D, Görlinger K, Haas T, Imberger G, Jacob M, Lancé M, Llau J, Mallett S, Meier J, Rahe-Meyer N, Samama CM, Smith A, Solomon C, Van der Linden P, Wikkelsø AJ, Wouters P, Wyffels P. Management of severe perioperative bleeding: guidelines from the European Society of Anaesthesiology. Eur J Anaesthesiol. 2013;30(6):270–382. https://doi.org/10.1097/EJA.0b013e32835f4d5b. Erratum in: Eur J Anaesthesiol 2014 Apr;31(4):247.
28. Society of Thoracic Surgeons Blood Conservation Guideline Task Force; Ferraris VA, Brown JR, Despotis GJ, Hammon JW, Reece TB, Saha SP, Song HK, Clough ER; Society of Cardiovascular Anesthesiologists Special Task Force on Blood Transfusion; Shore-Lesserson LJ, Goodnough LT, Mazer CD, Shander A, Stafford-Smith M, Waters J; International Consortium for Evidence Based Perfusion; Baker RA, Dickinson TA, FitzGerald DJ, Likosky DS, Shann KG. 2011 update to the Society of Thoracic Surgeons and the Society of

Cardiovascular Anesthesiologists blood conservation clinical practice guidelines. Ann Thorac Surg. 2011;91(3):944–82. https://doi.org/10.1016/j.athoracsur.2010.11.078.
29. Lelubre C, Vincent JL. Red blood cell transfusion in the critically ill patient. Ann Intensive Care. 2011;1:43. https://doi.org/10.1186/2110-5820-1-43.
30. Vallet B, Robin E, Lebuffe G. Venous oxygen saturation as a physiologic transfusion trigger. Crit Care. 2010;14(2):213. https://doi.org/10.1186/cc8854. Epub 2010 Mar 9
31. Hajjar LA, Vincent JL, Galas FR, Nakamura RE, Silva CM, Santos MH, Fukushima J, Kalil Filho R, Sierra DB, Lopes NH, Mauad T, Roquim AC, Sundin MR, Leão WC, Almeida JP, Pomerantzeff PM, Dallan LO, Jatene FB, Stolf NA, Auler JO Jr. Transfusion requirements after cardiac surgery: the TRACS randomized controlled trial. JAMA. 2010;304(14):1559–67. https://doi.org/10.1001/jama.2010.1446.
32. Ranucci M, Solomon C. Supplementation of fibrinogen in acquired bleeding disorders: experience, evidence, guidelines, and licences. Br J Anaesth. 2012;109(2):135–7. https://doi.org/10.1093/bja/aes227.
33. Kor DJ, Gajic O. blood product transfusion in the critical care setting. Curr Opin Crit Care. 2010;16:309–16.
34. Enriquez LJ, Shore-Lesserson L. Point-of-care coagulation testing and transfusion algorithms. Br J Anaesth. 2009;103(Suppl 1):i14–22. https://doi.org/10.1093/bja/aep318.
35. Camm AJ, Kirchhof P, Lip GY, Schotten U, Savelieva I, Ernst S, Van Gelder IC, Al-Attar N, Hindricks G, Prendergast B, Heidbuchel H, Alfieri O, Angelini A, Atar D, Colonna P, De Caterina R, De Sutter J, Goette A, Gorenek B, Heldal M, Hohloser SH, Kolh P, Le Heuzey JY, Ponikowski P, Rutten FH, ESC Committee for Practice Guidelines. Guidelines for the management of atrial fibrillation: the Task Force for the Management of Atrial Fibrillation of the European Society of Cardiology (ESC). Europace. 2010;12(10):1360–420. https://doi.org/10.1093/europace/euq350. Erratum in: Europace. 2011;13(7):1058. Dosage error in article text
36. Estes NA 3rd, Halperin JL, Calkins H, Ezekowitz MD, Gitman P, Go AS, McNamara RL, Messer JV, Ritchie JL, Romeo SJ, Waldo AL, Wyse DG, American College of Cardiology/American Heart Association Task Force on Performance Measures, Physician Consortium for Performance Improvement (Writing Committee to Develop Clinical Performance Measures for Atrial Fibrillation), Heart Rhythm Society. ACC/AHA/Physician Consortium 2008 clinical performance measures for adults with nonvalvular atrial fibrillation or atrial flutter: a report of the American College of Cardiology/American Heart Association Task Force on Performance Measures and the Physician Consortium for Performance Improvement (Writing Committee to Develop Clinical Performance Measures for Atrial Fibrillation): developed in collaboration with the Heart Rhythm Society. Circulation. 2008;117(8):1101–20. https://doi.org/10.1161/CIRCULATIONAHA.107.187192. Epub 2008 Feb 18
37. Dunning J, Treasure T, Versteegh M, Nashef SA, EACTS Audit and Guidelines Committee. Guidelines on the prevention and management of de novo atrial fibrillation after cardiac and thoracic surgery. Eur J Cardiothorac Surg. 2006;30(6):852–72. https://doi.org/10.1016/j.ejcts.2006.09.003. Epub 2006 Oct 27
38. Fernando HC, Jaklitsch MT, Walsh GL, Tisdale JE, Bridges CD, Mitchell JD, Shrager JB. The Society of Thoracic Surgeons practice guideline on the prophylaxis and management of atrial fibrillation associated with general thoracic surgery: executive summary. Ann Thorac Surg. 2011;92(3):1144–52.
39. Coppens M, Eikelboom JW, Hart RG, Yusuf S, Lip GY, Dorian P, Shestakovska O, Connolly SJ. The CHA2DS2-VASc score identifies those patients with atrial fibrillation and a CHADS2 score of 1 who are unlikely to benefit from oral anticoagulant therapy. Eur Heart J. 2013;34(3):170–6. https://doi.org/10.1093/eurheartj/ehs314. Epub 2012 Sep 27
40. Ley SJ, Koulakis D. Temporary pacing after cardiac surgery. AACN Adv Crit Care. 2015;26(3):275–80.
41. Cheng DC, David TE. Perioperative care in cardiac anesthesia and surgery. Lippincott Williams & Wilkins; 2006.

42. The Antiarrhythmics versus Implantable Defibrillators (AVID) Investigation. A comparison of anti-arrhythmic-drug therapy with implantable defibrillators in patients resuscitated from near-fatal ventricular arrhythmias. N Engl J Med. 1997;337:1576.
43. O'Collaghan PA, Ruskin JN. Current status of implantable cardioverter-defibrillator. Curr Probl Cardiol. 1997;22:641–707.
44. Edwards FH, Engelman RM, Houck P, Shahian DM, Bridges CR. The Society of Thoracic Surgeons practice guideline series: antibiotic prophylaxis in cardiac surgery, part I: duration. Ann Thorac Surg. 2006;81(1):397–404.
45. Bratzler DW, Houck PM, Workgroup SI. Antimicrobial prophylaxis for surgery: an advisory statement from the National Surgical Infection Prevention Project. Am J Surg. 2005;189(4):395–404.
46. Özker E, Saritaş B, Vuran C, Yörüker U, Ulugöl H, Türköz R. Delayed sternal closure after pediatric cardiac operations; single center experience: a retrospective study. J Cardiothorac Surg. 2012;7(1):102.
47. Dieberg G, Smart NA, King N. Minimally invasive cardiac surgery: a systematic review and meta-analysis. Int J Cardiol. 2016;223:554–60.
48. Griffiths MJ, Cordingley J, Price S, editors. Cardiovascular critical care. Wiley; 2011.
49. Nishimura RA, Otto CM, Bonow RO, Carabello BA, Erwin JP, Guyton RA, O'Gara PT, Ruiz CE, Skubas NJ, Sorajja P, Sundt TM. American College of Cardiology/American Heart Association task force on practice guidelines. 2014 aha/acc guideline for the management of patients with valvular heart disease: a report of the American College of Cardiology/American Heart Association Task Force on Practice Guidelines. J Am Coll Cardiol. 2014;63(22):2438–88.
50. Kiefer T, Park L, Tribouilloy C, Cortes C, Casillo R, Chu V, Delahaye F, Durante-Mangoni E, Edathodu J, Falces C, Logar M. Association between valvular surgery and mortality among patients with infective endocarditis complicated by heart failure. JAMA. 2011;306(20):2239–47.
51. Baddour LM, Wilson WR, Bayer AS, Fowler VG, Bolger AF, Levison ME, Ferrieri P, Gerber MA, Tani LY, Gewitz MH, Tong DC. Infective endocarditis. Circulation. 2005;111(23):e394–43.
52. Omar AS, Ewila H, Allam M, Aboulnagah S, Hanoura S, Sivadasan PC, Bilal O, Pattath AR, AlKhulaifi A. Improving incidence of postoperative atrial fibrillation after cardiac surgery using simplified clinical practice guidelines. J Intensive Care Med. 2016:0885066616679622.
53. Thygesen K, Alpert JS, White HD, Jaffe AS, Apple FS, Galvani M, Katus HA, Newby LK, Ravkilde J, Chaitman B, Clemmensen PM. Universal definition of myocardial infarction: Kristian Thygesen, Joseph S. Alpert and Harvey D. White on behalf of the Joint ESC/ACCF/AHA/WHF Task Force for the Redefinition of Myocardial Infarction. Eur Heart J. 2007;28(20):2525–38.
54. Omar AS, Sudarsanan S, Hanoura S, Osman H, Sivadasan PC, Shouman Y, Tuli AK, Singh R, Al Khulaifi A. Kinetics of highly sensitive troponin T after cardiac surgery. Biomed Res Int. 2015;2015
55. O'Neal JB, Shaw AD, Billings FT. Acute kidney injury following cardiac surgery: current understanding and future directions. Crit Care. 2016;20(1):187.
56. Mehta RL, Kellum JA, Shah SV, Molitoris BA, Ronco C, Warnock DG, Levin A. Acute Kidney Injury Network (AKIN): report of an initiative to improve outcomes in acute kidney injury. Crit Care. 2007;11(2):R31.

Postoperative Cardiac Surgical Pain Management

Moustafa Rezk, Ahmed Fayed ElGeziry,
and Nabil A. Shallik

1 Introduction

Pain after cardiac surgery is a common problem that requires prompt attention and effective management to avoid adverse outcomes. Approximately 30% to 75% of patients develop moderate to severe postoperative pain after cardiac surgery, which carries a massive burden on the health care system [1]. Uncontrolled pain in these population carries the risk of postoperative pulmonary infections, prolonged length of hospital stay, increased time to extubation, and the possibility of developing chronic persistent pain which affects the patient both socially and psychologically.

Despite advances in analgesic techniques, postoperative cardiac surgical pain remains difficult to manage.This is due to several factors including patient comorbidities that may limit treatment options, as well as variables such as age, gender, the complexity and duration of the surgery, and the presence of pain at multiple postoperative sites.

Historically, large doses of opioids were used to manage pain in cardiac surgery patients. However this approach came with significant side effects such as respiratory depression, nausea, and vomiting, studies have shown that more than 30% of patients experience opioid-related adverse effects during hospitalization, and 5% to 10% of previously opioid naïve patients may become new persistent opioid users [2, 3].

With the adoption of fast track protocols, multimodal analgesia has become the cornerstone of postoperative pain management. This approach facilitates shorter

M. Rezk · A. F. ElGeziry
Hamad Medical Corporation, Doha, Qatar

N. A. Shallik (✉)
Clinical Anaesthesiology Department, College of Medicine Qatar University
and Weill Cornell Medical College, Doha, Qatar
e-mail: Nshallik@hamad.qa

E. Elmistekawy, N. A. Shallik (eds.), *Perioperative Care of Cardiac Surgery Patients*, https://doi.org/10.1007/978-3-032-09817-7_4

extubation times, reduced hospital stays, fewer opoid-related side effects, and overall lower morbidity.

Nowadays, many analgesic modalities have been developed including conservative approaches such as opioid sparing medications and locoregional techniques. However no single modality has yet been proven to be the most effective for acute pain relief.

1.1 Pathophysiology

As with any type of surgery, cardiac surgery causes tissue disruption and stimulates an inflammatory response. This tissue disruption includes skin incision, sternotomy, rib retraction, chest drain placement, and site of vein graft harvesting. Postoperative pain in cardiac surgery is a type of acute pain which follows the same classical four phases of pain pathway it begins by the release of inflammatory mediators at the site of surgical manipulation that elicits an action potential wthis is called transduction which is then transmitted via sensory pathways to the dorsal horn of the spinal cord until reaching the somatosensory cortex a phase called central perception and finally the pain is modulated via endogenous opioids to reduce the intensity of the perceived pain. It is crucial to understand this pathway as different analgesic modalities aim to block the pain at various phases. Also, it is very important to exclude residual ischemia or incomplete revascularization as potential causes of postoperative pain which are not uncommon factors in pain generation after cardiac surgery.

1.2 Factors Contributing to Postoperative Cardiac Surgical Pain

Pain after cardiac surgery can originate from multiple sources, and is typically most severe during the first two to three postoperative days, one of the most common sources of pain is the sternotomy including sternal retraction and rib injuries.

The site of mediastinal and pleural drains, as well as internal mammary artery (IMA) dissection is another source of pain. All these factors contribute to chest pain, which is the most frequently reported type of pain following surgery. However we should not ignore other types of pain like leg pain in patients undergoing saphenous venous grafting, which is not uncommon. It often becomes more noticeable after the third postoperative day due to decrease in chest pain which unmasks the leg pain. Sometimes shoulder pain can be caused by intraoperative positioning such as the lateral decubitus position.

Other factors such as gender and age also influence the severity of postoperative pain. Women tend to experience more severe pain than men, and individuals under the age of 60 generally report more pain than older patients.The longer the duration of the surgery and the more complex the procedure, the more pain will be elicited postoperatively. All these factors should be acknowledged to develop effective, individualized pain management strategies [4].

1.3 Chronic Postsurgical Pain

One of the most debilitating complications following cardiac surgery, is the development of chronic postoperative pain, its incidence varies between 20% and 55% it is defined as pain that persists for more than 3 months after surgery. This complication has a significant negative impact on patients' lives socially, psychologically, and economically [4]. It most commonly in two forms chronic chest pain and chronic leg pain.

The best approach to managing this condition is prevention, primarily through adequate control of acute postoperative pain. There are a lot of precipitating factors that aggravate this condition like preoperative or postoperative psychological vulnerability, redo surgeries, severe acute postoperative pain, non-elective operations, the increased need for analgesic use in the early postoperative period, and longer duration of surgery and its complexity.

Chronic chest pain is most often neuropathic in origin. It results from different mechanisms like intercostal nerve damage, IMA harvesting, disruption of the costochondral junction, brachial plexus injury, rib fractures, sternal infection, and surgical scar formation.

Chronic leg pain often presenting as neuralgia should not be ignored, especially in cases where saphenous vein harvesting is performed during CABG surgery.

2 Different Analgesic Modalities for Postoperative Pain Management

Many analgesic modalities are continuously emerging for pain management after cardiac surgery; however, no single modality has been proven to be the most effective in relieving pain, as each method has its own advantages and disadvantages. But with the adoption of fast track protocols, multimodal analgesia has proven to be highly effective in controlling pain.

We can broadly divide the analgesic modalities into pharmacological and non-pharmacological approaches, pharmacological methods can be further categorized into systemic medications and locoregional techniques.

Non- pharmacological methods can be in the form of behavioral therapy, acupuncture, and other supportive interventions.

2.1 Systemic Medications

In the past, opioids were the primary method of analgesic method in pain management for cardiac surgery, but many side effects were reported like nausea, vomiting, and respiratory depression, these adverse effects often delayed the extubation time and prolonged hospitalization negatively impacting patient health and negatively and the overall health care system. Nowadays we are in the era of fast track and Enhanced Recovery After Cardiac Surgery (ERAC) protocols which have been applied successfully to the cardiac surgery due to the adoption of multimodal analgesia and the use of opioid sparing medications. In the following sections, we will explore different medications and explain their postoperative effects.

2.1.1 Opioids

Opioids remain the cornerstone of postoperative pain management in cardiac surgery, despite their known side effects.We use opioid sparing but not opioid free analgesics postoperatively which means that opioids still have a crucial role in pain control. There are different types of opioids, but studies have not shown the superiority of one over another.

Intravenous (IV) morphine has been assessed in three studies, all of which showed decreased pain scores without increased side effects. Postoperative use of morphine improves patient satisfaction and decreases acute pain [5].

One randomized controlled trail (RCT) study in 2004 compared the use of patient controlled analgesia (PCA) morphine alone with PCA morphine plus background IV infusion in patients extubated after CABG surgery, Opioid consumption increased but pain relief improved without increased side effects. Nurse-administrated subcutaneous morphine is another method that can be used. Both groups were compared with no statistical difference between them, both methods were satisfactory for the patients. There was debate regarding the use of remifentanil as it can induce opioid hyperalgesia, but studies showed no difference in efficacy between PCA remifentanil and PCA morphine [5, 6].

Oral oxycodone has been found to be an effective treatment in comparison to IV morphine even after extremely painful procedures.

Morphine can be administrated intravenously 5 mg every 4 to 6 hours according to NRS score; PCA morphine bolus dose 1 mg and lock out time is 10 minutes.

Oxycodone dose is 5 mg orally four times daily.

2.1.2 Paracetamol

Paracetamol has long been used as part of a multimodal analgesia approach. It is not a classic NSAID, rather it works through a central mechanism to provide mild to moderate anti-inflammatory effects. Many studies have not demonstrated a significant reduction in opioid consumption when using paracetamol alone, However it has been found to be more effective when used as a part of a multimodal analgesic regimen. The recommended dose is 1000 mg administered intravenously or orally up to four times daily [4, 5].

2.1.3 NSAID

These drugs are non-steroidal anti-inflammatory drugs (NSAID) which act via inhibition of the cyclooxygenase (COX) enzyme, leading to reduced prostaglandin synthesis. There are broadly two classes, non-selective COX inhibitors and selective $COX\text{-}_2$ inhibitors, which emerged as alternative to reduce the unwanted side effects of non-selective COX inhibitors such as gastrointestinal (GI) upset. However, COX_2 inhibitors have still been associated with certain cardiovascular complications.

There has been ongoing debate regarding the use of NSAID in the postoperative period due to the potential risk of bleeding. However one retrospective study was on ketorolac a non-selective COX inhibitor, analyzed data from 488 patients who received ketorolac within 72 hours after CABG surgery. Postoperative bleeding, renal injury, hemorrhage requiring reoperation, and perioperative cardiovascular complications were assessed. No significant difference were found compared to the control group in terms of gastrointestinal bleeding or need for reoperation due to hemorrhage [1]. Ketorolac can be administered as a single 30 mg intravenous dose or every 6 hours if needed, not exceeding a total daily dose of 120 mg.

Many other studies have shown the safety of NSAID in terms of GI and renal side effects along with improved pain control and reduced opioid consumption, However some studies have suggested that selective COX_2 inhibitors may increase the risk of sternal wound infections when used continuously for 14 days [7]. In summary, NSAID are generally safe to use postoperatively and are effective in reducing opioid consumption and managing pain. However, further research is needed to better understand the safety profile of selective COX_2 inhibitors [7]. Diclofenac can be given orally 50 mg three times daily, and celecoxib at 200 mg orally twice daily.

2.1.4 Magnesium Sulphate

Magnesium exerts its analgesic effects by antagonizing calcium and NMDA receptors. Some studies have shown that postoperative magnesium infusion can reduce pain scores, but it should still be used with caution, as it can cause bradycardia, hypotension, and asystole [4].

Magnesium can be initiated intraoperatively with a bolus dose of 50 mg/kg, followed by a continuous infusion at 15 mg/kg/hr.

2.1.5 Dexmetomidine

Dexmedetomidine is an alpha-2 adrenergic agonist that causes sedation, anxiolysis, and sympatholysis through the stimulation of alpha-2 receptors located in the locus coeruleus and spinal cord. It is widely used in the ICU as a postoperative sedative.

Dexmedetomidine has been studied as an infusion agent compared to placebo, both intraoperatively and for 12 hours postoperatively. Results showed a reduction in pain scores, shorter time to extubation, and decreased opioid consumption. Another study compared it to morphine, and no significant difference was observed between the two groups, except for a greater decrease in heart rate with dexmedetomidine [7].

Dexmedetomidine is a good choice for postoperative analgesia and generally does not compromise hemodynamic stability, but close monitoring is still required, as prolonged infusion can lead to hypotension and bradycardia.

It is administered as a continuous infusion at 0.5 μg/kg/hr, starting from the initiation of anesthesia and continuing until tracheal extubation in the ICU.

2.1.6 Ketamine

Ketamine is an NMDA receptor antagonist that acts through dissociative anesthesia, producing a combination of hallucinations, analgesia, catalepsy, and amnesia.

Many studies have not shown a significant difference in pain scores compared to opioids, although it is often used as part of a multimodal analgesic regimen. Ketamine does not cause respiratory depression, and the use of the S-ketamine isomer has been associated with fewer side effects [4].

2.1.7 Gabapentin and Pregabalin

Both gabapentin and pregabalin are used as neuromodulatory medications. They function as gamma-aminobutyric acid (GABA) analogs that act on dorsal horn cells to reduce neuronal hyperexcitability, central sensitization, and wind-up phenomena.

Studies have shown mixed results. Some have demonstrated a reduction in opioid consumption when these drugs are used in non-cardiac surgeries, but results regarding postoperative pain in cardiac surgery remain debatable. They are mainly used in chronic pain management rather than acute postoperative pain [1].

Pregabalin can be administered 2 hours prior to surgery at a dose of 300 mg, and gabapentin at 1200 mg. Postoperatively, pregabalin can be given at 150 mg twice daily, and gabapentin at 600 mg three times daily.

2.2 Locoregional Techniques

Over the last decade, regional analgesia has progressed tremendously with the emergence of new fascial plane blocks that help reduce postoperative pain while avoiding the side effects of medications. These blocks are used as part of a multimodal analgesia regimen, which helps patients achieve faster recovery after cardiac surgery.

2.2.1 Thoracic Epidural Analgesia and Intrathecal Opioids

Thoracic epidural analgesia (TEA) has long been considered the gold standard for regional analgesia in cardiac surgery. In such procedures, it is essential to provide analgesia for surgical sites like sternotomy, thoracotomy, and chest tube incisions, which are innervated by the thoracic nerves (T1–T11). These nerves can be blocked using local anesthetics administered via the epidural space.

Studies have demonstrated multiple beneficial effects of TEA, including a reduction in respiratory complications, supraventricular arrhythmias, and myocardial infarction (MI). TEA also contributes to improved pain scores, shorter time to extubation, reduced opioid consumption, and a mild reduction in stress-induced hyperglycemia.

However, TEA is still not widely used, primarily due to the frequent systemic heparinization during cardiac surgeries and the common use of antiplatelet therapy, which raise concerns about the development of epidural hematoma—a serious and potentially devastating complication [1, 2, 5].

Nevertheless, some studies have shown that the risk of epidural hematoma after catheter placement for cardiac surgery is similar to that observed in general surgery.

Intrathecal opioids represent another option for analgesia. Intrathecal morphine is typically administered before general anesthesia, and some studies have shown that a dose of 5 mcg/kg can significantly reduce opioid consumption for up to 48 hours.

It also carries a minimal risk of spinal hematoma, although side effects such as pruritus, nausea, vomiting, and respiratory depression may occur and should be closely monitored during the early postoperative period [2].

2.2.2 Paravertebral Block (PVB)

Paravertebral block (PVB) is one of the regional analgesic techniques performed by injecting local anesthetics into the paravertebral space, lateral to where the spinal nerve roots emerge from the intervertebral foramina in the thoracic region. Its efficacy depends on the volume of injectate and the number of levels covered.

PVB provides excellent pain relief when administered unilaterally for thoracotomy incisions, while bilateral paravertebral block is required for median sternotomy. It offers the advantage of a lower risk of hypotension and epidural hematoma compared to thoracic epidural analgesia (TEA).

Some studies have shown that paravertebral catheters inserted at the end of surgery under direct visualization by the surgical team provide favorable pain scores at rest and during coughing over the first 72 hours. Additionally, functional expired volume and ambient air oxygen saturation improved compared to the TEA group at 24, 48, and 72 hours, with no reported incidence of pruritus, nausea, urinary retention, or postural hypotension [1].

Another study showed that patients who received bilateral PVB required less intraoperative fentanyl and were more likely to be extubated intraoperatively or immediately postoperatively. Bilateral paravertebral block offers pain control comparable to TEA, with fewer side effects [2].

2.2.3 Erector Spinae Plane Block

This type of block involves the injection of local anesthetics into the plane between the erector spinae muscles and the transverse process, lateral to the spine. It is considered a relatively new technique that is increasingly used following cardiac surgery.

It provides analgesia by covering the ipsilateral nerve distribution distal to the site of injection. Several studies have shown that it reduces opioid consumption, and it can be continued postoperatively via catheter insertion.

Compared to the paravertebral block, the ESP block poses a lower risk of hypotension, spinal hematoma, and pneumothorax. A large volume of injectate (20–30 mL) is required to achieve effective analgesia, due to the distance between the injection site and the target neural structures.

Studies in live patients have demonstrated that the injectate spreads along the ventral rami, the craniocaudal plane, and the lateral cutaneous branches of the intercostal nerves, providing enhanced and effective analgesia after cardiac surgery [2, 8].

2.2.4 Serratus Anterior (Deep and Superficial) Plane Block

This type of block can be performed either *superficial to the serratus anterior muscle* or *deep to it*, between the muscle and the *rib periosteum*. It is particularly suitable for *lateral chest wall incisions*, making it ideal for use in *thoracotomy procedures*.

Its role has been highlighted in minimally invasive cardiac surgeries, where it has been shown to *reduce pain scores and opioid consumption*. Its efficacy is *comparable to that of an intercostal nerve block*, but due to *reduced local vascularity*, the analgesic effect tends to *last longer* [2].

2.2.5 Parasternal Intercostal (Deep and Superficial) Plane Block

This group of blocks is collectively referred to as parasternal blocks. They involve injection of local anesthetics lateral to the sternum, either between the pectoralis major and intercostal muscles or deep between the intercostal muscles and the transversus thoracis muscle.

These blocks must be performed bilaterally to be effective, and their analgesic effect is primarily limited to the sternotomy incision. Multiple randomized controlled trials have shown that parasternal blocks improve pain scores and reduce opioid consumption. Both pre-incisional and post-incisional techniques are comparable in terms of postoperative pain relief [2].

Studies have shown that both superficial and deep parasternal blocks provide effective analgesia, with no clear superiority between them. Therefore, the superficial block is often preferred due to its lower risk profile while maintaining similar efficacy.

One theoretical risk associated with the deep block is injury to the internal mammary artery (IMA). This risk arises because the transversus thoracis is a thin muscle, and the IMA runs just inferior to its border. This is especially important in coronary artery bypass grafting (CABG), where the IMA is commonly used as a conduit.

2.3 Non-pharmacological Modalities

Other non-pharmacological modalities may also play a role in reducing pain after cardiac surgery, although further studies are needed. Several techniques have been investigated, including massage therapy, acupuncture, relaxation techniques, and behavioral modification.

Psychological status may influence pain intensity. In a survey of 197 patients scheduled to undergo coronary artery bypass graft (CABG) surgery, conducted 4 weeks preoperatively and 8 weeks postoperatively, a significant correlation was found between greater optimism and lower pain scores 2 months after surgery. The study concluded that positive expectations may promote better recovery. Optimism has also been associated with lower levels of proinflammatory cytokines, such as C-reactive protein and interleukin-6 (IL-6) [1].

Acupuncture has historically been recognized as an alternative therapy for managing various painful conditions. More recently, it has been studied in the context of cardiac surgery, with some studies suggesting that it may help reduce postoperative pain. However, the current evidence is limited, and additional research is needed to confirm its efficacy [9].

3 Conclusion

Effective control of postoperative pain in cardiac surgery is a crucial component of enhanced recovery protocols and is essential for preventing various short- and long-term complications that may impact patient health.

A Multimodal analgesic regimen is typically implemented, as no single technique has yet been proven to provide optimal pain relief. Therefore analgesic strategies must be tailored to each patient's condition in order to achieve maximum benefit.

References

1. Bigeleisen PE, Goehner N. Novel approaches in pain management in cardiac surgery. Curr Opin Anaesthesiol. 2015;28(1):89–94. https://doi.org/10.1097/ACO.0000000000000147. PMID: 25500688.
2. Grant MC, Gregory AJ, Ouanes JP. Regional analgesia for cardiac surgery. Curr Opin Anaesthesiol. 2022;35(5):605–12. https://doi.org/10.1097/ACO.0000000000001169. Epub 2022 Jul 27. PMID: 35900740.
3. Makkad B, Heinke TL, Sheriffdeen R, Khatib D, Brodt JL, Meng ML, Grant MC, Kachulis B, Popescu WM, Wu CL, Bollen BA. Practice advisory for preoperative and intraoperative pain management of cardiac surgical patients: part 2. Anesth Analg. 2023;137(1):26–47. https://doi.org/10.1213/ANE.0000000000006506. Epub 2023 Jun 16. PMID: 37326862.
4. Dabbagh A. Postoperative critical care for adult cardiac surgical patients. 2018. ISBN: 978-3-319-75746.
5. Bignami E, Castella A, Pota V, Saglietti F, Scognamiglio A, Trumello C, Pace MC, Allegri M. Perioperative pain management in cardiac surgery: a systematic review. Minerva Anestesiol. 2018;84(4):488–503. https://doi.org/10.23736/S0375-9393.17.12142-5. Epub 2017 Oct 12. PMID: 29027773.
6. Nachiyunde B, Lam L. The efficacy of different modes of analgesia in postoperative pain management and early mobilization in postoperative cardiac surgical patients: a systematic review. Ann Card Anaesth. 2018;21(4):363–70. https://doi.org/10.4103/aca.ACA_186_17. PMID: 30333328; PMCID: PMC6206788.
7. Maeßen T, Korir N, Van de Velde M, Kennes J, PogatzkPROSPECT Working Group of the European Society of Regional Anaesthesia and Pain Therapy. Pain management after cardiac surgery via median sternotomy: a systematic review with procedure-specific postoperative pain management (PROSPECT) recommendations. Eur J Anaesthesiol. 2023;40(10):758–68. https://doi.org/10.1097/EJA.0000000000001881. Epub 2023 Jul 19. PMID: 37501517.
8. Kelava M, Alfirevic A, Bustamante S, Hargrave J, Marciniak D. Regional anesthesia in cardiac surgery: an overview of fascial plane chest wall blocks. Anesth Analg. 2020;131(1):127–35. https://doi.org/10.1213/ANE.0000000000004682. PMID: 32032103.
9. Roshanzamir S, Haririan Y, Ghaderpanah R, Jahromi LSM, Dabbaghmanesh A. Investigation of the effects of acupuncture on post-operative chest pain after open heart surgery. J Acupunct Meridian Stud. 2023;16(4):133–8. https://doi.org/10.51507/j.jams.2023.16.4.133. PMID: 37609768.

Post-Cardiac Operations Wound Care

Rashad Alfkey, Hesham Aljohary,
and Mosab Ahmed Murad

1 Historical Overview

Julian et al. introduced the median sternotomy incision for heart surgery for the first time in 1957 [1]. Nevertheless, initial reports of a 5% infection rate that resulted in sternal dehiscence and heart exposure hampered its acceptability. Lee et al. showed how to successfully use omentum to close an open mediastinal defect in 1976. After this, patients who did not respond to first treatment were successfully treated with sternectomy followed by closure of the muscle flap or omental flap by Jurkiewicz et al. in 1977.

Pectoralis major, rectus abdominis, and latissimus dorsi are a few examples of pedicled muscle flaps that have been used over time to treat complex wounds. When it comes to treating infected sternal wounds, these flaps gained popularity as an alternative to omentum, which decreased the mortality rate [2].

R. Alfkey (✉)
Surgery Department, Hamad Medical Corporation, Doha, Qatar

Surgery Department, Weill Cornell Medical College in Qatar, Doha, Qatar

Surgery Department, Alazhar Faculty of Medicine, Cairo, Egypt
e-mail: rabdelmoaty@hamad.qa

H. Aljohary
Surgery Department, Hamad Medical Corporation, Doha, Qatar

Surgery Department, Weill Cornell Medical College in Qatar, Doha, Qatar

M. A. Murad
Surgery Department, Hamad Medical Corporation, Doha, Qatar

E. Elmistekawy, N. A. Shallik (eds.), *Perioperative Care of Cardiac Surgery Patients*, https://doi.org/10.1007/978-3-032-09817-7_5

2 Surgical Site Infections (SSI)

SSIs after heart surgery still carry a substantial risk. Sternal wound infections (SWIs) are associated with greater rates of morbidity, death, longer hospital stays, and higher expenses; they affect about 8.49% of sternotomies [3]. Studies reveal that hospital stays for sternal infection patients are usually three times longer than for noninfected patients [4].

Sternal wound infections (SWIs) can vary in severity, ranging from superficial to deep infections. Superficial Sternal Wound Infections (SSWI) involve the skin, subcutaneous tissue, and pectoralis fascia. The incidence of SSWI is reported to be between 0.5% and 8%, with associated morbidity and mortality rates ranging from 0.5% to 9%. Symptoms of SSWI typically include pain, tenderness, swelling, redness, heat, and purulent discharge, while the sternum remains stable. Fortunately, these infections can often be effectively treated with intravenous antibiotics and local wound care [5].

Deep sternal wound infection (DSWI) is a serious complication that involves infections beneath the subcutaneous tissue, bone, or cartilage, as well as the mediastinal space (mediastinitis), which can lead to sternal dehiscence and potentially expose the heart [6]. DSWI is one of the most complex and devastating complications following median sternotomy, significantly affecting patient prognosis and hospital budgets, with in-hospital mortality rates ranging from 7% to 35% [7] The incidence of DSWI remains significant, ranging between 0.5% and 6.8%, with in-hospital mortality rates between 7% and 47%. Excess costs are mainly attributed to antibiotic treatments, surgical procedures, and prolonged hospital stays [8]. Diagnosing DSWI requires evidence of infection, sternal instability during surgical reexploration, and positive culture results from surgical sites or the mediastinal area [9]. Studies have shown that patients who develop DSWI have a lower survival rate compared to those who do not. For example, Filsou et al. found a 15% reduction in absolute survival for patients with DSWI by the end of the first year [10]. In a 10-year follow-up study after coronary artery bypass grafting, the adjusted survival rate was 39% for patients who developed DSWI compared to 70% for those who did not [11].

3 Types of SWI

There are various classifications for sternal wound infections, leading to inconsistencies in current wound reconstruction techniques. One of the most widely used classifications is the Pairolero and Arnold Classification of Deep Sternal Wound Infections (DSWI) established in 1984 [12]. This classification system was created to facilitate the timely diagnosis and effective management of sternal wound infections. It divides SWI into three types based on the timing of clinical presentation:

Type I infections typically occur within the first month after cardiac surgery, characterized by a serous drainage from the sternal wound without any signs of osteomyelitis, costochondritis, or mediastinal suppuration.

Type II infections manifest within the first few weeks after sternotomy, presenting with purulent drainage, wire exposure, sternal osteomyelitis, mediastinitis, and occasionally costochondritis.

Type III infections involve a chronically draining sinus tract into the sternum or costochondral arches, typically developing several months after the initial cardiac surgery.

4 Microbiology

Postoperative infections may arise from commensal skin bacteria that penetrate deeper layers following wound dehiscence, which exposes underlying tissues. Obtaining a bacterial culture from wound secretions is crucial for developing selecting optimum antibiotic therapy, wound classification, and treatment plans. Cultures of purulent exudates can be collected from surgical wounds or from the mediastinum during surgery or by needle aspiration of the anterior mediastinal.

Staphylococcus epidermidis is a common cause of poststernotomy mediastinitis, particularly when foreign materials like prosthetic heart valves are involved. Around 75% of *Staphylococcus epidermidis* strains are resistant to methicillin. On the other hand, *Staphylococcus aureus* has been increasingly linked to colonization of patients' nasal passages.

According to the National Nosocomial Infections Surveillance System, the prevalence of MRSA has surged from 30% in 1989 to 60% in 2005 among ICU patients with nosocomial infections. MRSA was identified as the primary microorganism in a third of patients with DSWI [29–35]. In their study, Al-Majid et al. discovered that Methicillin-Sensitive *Staphylococcus aureus* (MSSA) is commonly found in male diabetic patients who have undergone Coronary Artery Bypass Grafting (CABG) surgery. Other organisms that have been implicated include *Escherichia coli*, Enterobacter species, *Pseudomonas aeruginosa*, β-hemolytic streptococci, *Enterococcus faecalis*, *Proteus mirabilis*, *Klebsiella pneumoniae*, and *Serratia marcescens* [17, 36].

5 Risk Factors for Sternal Wound Infection (SWI)

These can be categorized into patient-related, intraoperative, and postoperative factors. It is crucial to implement various preoperative preventive strategies to mitigate the risk of developing this serious complication. Failure to address these risk factors can lead to potentially catastrophic consequences.

Patient-related risk factors include age, female gender, obesity, diabetes mellitus, smoking, alcoholism, malignancy, steroid therapy, presence of comorbidities, *Staphylococcus aureus* nasal carriage, skin infections, osteoporosis, chronic infections (such as HIV, hepatitis B, hepatitis C, or bacterial infections lasting longer than 4 weeks, or being on antibiotics at the time of surgery), and emergent/urgent surgery [13].

Intraoperative risk factors include undergoing coronary artery bypass grafting along with valve or aortic surgery, prolonged duration of aortic cross-clamp, cardiopulmonary bypass perfusion for an extended period, using both internal mammary arteries, employing bone wax, extensive electrocauterization, needing prosthetic implants, utilizing an intra-aortic balloon pump or ventricular assist device, experiencing postoperative bleeding, and requiring transfusions.

Postoperative risk factors may include the need for prolonged ventilator and inotropic support, reexploration for bleeding, postoperative transfusions, and an extended stay in the intensive care unit (ICU) [7, 8, 10].

There is a range of findings regarding the influence of gender on Deep Surgical Wound Infection (DSWI) following surgery. While some studies have indicated a higher incidence of DSWI in male patients, others have reported a higher incidence in female patients [14, 15]. On the other hand, the risk of SSIs increases with age, as older individuals often have reduced tissue regeneration capabilities and may be affected by underlying systemic diseases. Consequently, older patients may experience delayed wound healing and are more susceptible to infections [16].

Numerous published studies have confirmed the significance of obesity and diabetes mellitus as risk factors for DSWI [13, 17]. Prolonged tissue hyperglycemia can lead to the accumulation of advanced glycation end products, disturbances in microcirculation, inadequate oxygen supply to tissues, increased apoptosis of repair cells, and dysfunction in metabolic and immune system defenses. These factors collectively contribute to an elevated risk of infection and delayed wound healing. Animal studies have shown that diabetic mice exhibit increased sugar content in skin tissue, which is directly correlated with delayed wound healing following skin incisions. Notably, hyperglycemia and associated lesions have been found to impair the molecular regulation of hypoxia-related genes (HIF1A), while upregulating genes responsible for extracellular matrix formation [18].

Prolonged smoking has been shown to have detrimental effects on the immune system. It can lower the concentration of immunoglobulin, inhibit the activity of lysozyme, decrease the number of NK cells, CD3+, CD4+, and CD8+ T cells, ultimately compromising immune function. Furthermore, smoking can lead to respiratory edema, increased sputum production, pulmonary infections, and even chronic obstructive pulmonary disease (COPD) [19]. The frequent coughing resulting from COPD can cause repeated friction at the site of a sternum fracture leading to elevated pressure on the steel wire, raising the likelihood of both sternal cracking and steel wire fracture [20].

Renal insufficiency is often accompanied by malnutrition, anemia, and decreased immunity, increasing the risk of infection, and delaying wound healing. Additionally, it places added strain on the heart, diminishes the patient's surgical tolerance, and impairs the effectiveness of debridement procedures [21].

Malnutrition can lead to inadequate protein synthesis and a decrease in red blood cell count. This can slow down cell regeneration and impair the function of inflammatory and immune cells, making the body more susceptible to infections. Additionally, malnutrition can hinder the formation of granulation tissue and collagen fibers, ultimately delaying the healing process of wounds [22].

The internal mammary artery (IMA) grafts, particularly when used on both sides, have been linked to a higher risk of SSIs. Different methods for harvesting IMA grafts exist. The skeletonization harvest technique is recognized for significantly decreasing the occurrence of deep sternal wound infections (DSWI), especially in diabetic and obese patients, due to its superior preservation of collateral sternal flow and internal thoracic veins. Nevertheless, some cardiothoracic surgeons are hesitant to adopt this method due to concerns about potential damage to the graft conduit [23].

Prolonged durations of cardiopulmonary bypass time and aortic cross-clamp time, along with the use of an intra-aortic balloon pump, have been associated with an increased risk of infection in certain cases. Additionally, postoperative bleeding, the need for reoperation, and sternal rewiring have been identified as contributing factors. The type of sternal saw used during the procedure and the application of bone wax have also been recognized as potential risk factors [24].

The utilization of bone wax has been associated with an elevated risk of DSWI in animal studies. Nevertheless, a prospective, randomized trial involving 400 patients revealed no adverse effects [7].

6 Antimicrobial Prophylaxis

The benefits of proper antimicrobial prophylaxis for patients undergoing cardiac surgery have been established. However, there is still ongoing debate surrounding the choice of antibiotic, dosage, duration, serum and tissue levels, and timing of antimicrobial prophylaxis. According to the Society of Thoracic Surgeons Practice Guidelines, it is recommended that cephalosporin be administered within 60 minutes of the skin incision and continued for 24–72 hours [7, 9, 38]. First-generation cephalosporins such as cefazolin, second-generation cephalosporins like cefamandole and cefuroxime, and third generation cephalosporins such as cefotaxime have all been shown to effectively reduce SSIs in cardiac surgery. According to Engelman et al., vancomycin is typically recommended for patients with a history of type I allergic reactions to β-lactam agents or in cases where there is a high incidence of MRSA within the institution [38, 44].

The timing of prophylactic antimicrobial administration remains controversial. According to the 2011 American College of Cardiology/American Heart Association guidelines for cardiac surgery, it is recommended that antibiotic prophylaxis be initiated 30 to 60 minutes before surgery [7, 39, 40–42]. Factors such as the use of cardiopulmonary bypass, hypothermia, the duration of the operation, high mortality rates, and the costs associated with deep sternal wound infections (DSWI) suggest that prolonging antimicrobial prophylaxis in cardiac surgery may be beneficial. A 2011 systematic review and meta-analysis of the literature supported longer-term antimicrobial prophylaxis of more than 24 hours in these patients [7]. Additionally, research by Lador et al. indicated that a shorter duration of prophylaxis (24 hours or less) was linked to higher rates of DSWI, surgical intervention for various surgical site infections (SSI), and endocarditis. However, there was no significant difference in outcomes between 48 hours of prophylaxis and longer durations [7, 43].

Some studies have emphasized the significance of weight-based antibiotic dosing in obese patients, as well as the necessity for multiple doses during extended procedures (lasting more than two half-lives of the drug) or in the event of significant blood loss during the procedure. Additionally, researchers have found that administering a cefazolin bolus followed by continuous infusion can enhance pharmacokinetic and pharmacodynamic parameters, resulting in improved drug concentrations in the cardiac muscle [7, 45].

7 Prevention of Surgical Site Infection

Preventing postoperative infections ensures a successful patient's recovery and involves implementing good hygiene practices, administering antibiotics before and after surgery, and closely observing the patient. Reducing the bioburden around the incision during the postoperative period can significantly decrease the risk of infection. It is recommended to obtain nasal swabs from all patients before the procedure and administer intranasal mupirocin along with a chlorhexidine bath the night before surgery. Prophylactic antibiotics should also be given to further prevent infections.

If a patient is suspected of having an infection before elective surgery, it is important to identify and treat the source before proceeding with the operation. Elective surgery should be postponed until the infection has been resolved. Optimizing the patient's nutritional status and controlling their blood sugar levels are also vital in reducing the risk of infection [37]. Basic preventive measures, include minimizing preoperative hospitalization, enhancing oxygenation during the perioperative period, preoperative cleansing with an antiseptic solution, hair removal using scissors or depilatory cream rather than shaving, and scrubbing the operation site with an appropriate antiseptic solution followed by allowing it to dry. Antiseptic solutions such as chlorhexidine, alcohol, or povidone-iodine can be utilized, as the CDC guidelines do not favor one over the others [7, 9].

8 Patient Evaluation

The initial evaluation of a patient involves a thorough examination of their medical history and a physical assessment. It is crucial to review any previous sternotomy procedures and the use of internal mammary arteries for cardiac revascularization. Additionally, risk factors such as diabetes, obesity, and chronic obstructive airway disease should be carefully evaluated. During the physical examination, special attention should be given to assessing the wound, wound drainage, wire exposure, sternal instability, and the possibility of communication with the pleural space. An elevated leukocyte count is typically observed, and close monitoring of renal function is essential as its decline may indicate the onset of multisystem organ failure. Needle aspiration of collections can provide bacteriologic evidence of deep infection in a superficial wound that is healing, with underlying sternal bone dehiscence.

It is important to rule out other potential causes of sepsis, such as abdominal sepsis from mesenteric infarction and empyema of the gall bladder. By conducting a thorough patient evaluation, healthcare providers can ensure accurate diagnosis and appropriate treatment for the patient's condition.

9 Radiologic Evaluation

Plain chest radiographs are valuable for identifying empyema and pleural effusions, while a chest CT examination and magnetic resonance imaging can aid in detecting substernal fluid collections. X-rays and CT scans may reveal mediastinal widening, mediastinal gas-liquid level, mediastinal emphysema, pleural effusion, and wire displacement [25]. It is recommended that each patient undergo a chest CT examination before debridement to assess sternum stability, facilitate a more thorough debridement process, and prepare for subsequent wound closure treatment. However, it is important to note that a CT examination alone may not be sufficient. Studies have shown that CT has limitations in identifying costochondritis. Additionally, cardiac surgery patients often have metal internal fixators, making MRI unsuitable for soft tissue imaging. Research has indicated that PET/CT has higher sensitivity and specificity compared to CT. By utilizing PET/CT, clinicians can reduce their reliance on radiologists and decrease the likelihood of missed diagnoses [26–28].

10 Treatment of Sternal Wound Infections (SWI)

Treatment involves infection control, general drainage, wound reconstruction, and the treatment of sternal instability/defect [25]. Aggressive debridement and muscle transposition are the preferred treatment options for most patients with infected median sternotomy wounds. The management of SWI needs a multidisciplinary approach. Key components of treatment include early surgical debridement, Negative Pressure Wound Therapy (NPWT), and antibiotic therapy, effective local dressings, and closely monitoring systemic parameters and overall nutrition.

11 Antibiotic Therapy

The initial antibiotic therapy regimen is determined based on a direct examination of Gram-staining. Vancomycin is administered when Gram-positive cocci (GPC) are identified, while β-lactams are administered when Gram-negative bacteria (GNB) are identified. If Gram-staining is inconclusive, both β-lactams and vancomycin are administered. The choice of β-lactams depends on host factors, such as the risk for infection with antibiotic-resistant pathogens and observed local susceptibility patterns. This therapy is then adjusted as needed based on the antibiograms of suspected causative microorganisms. Antibiotic therapy is continued for 6 weeks after the last surgical debridement [46, 47].

Identification of the microorganisms responsible for DSWIs is crucial when deciding on the appropriate antimicrobial treatment. Systemic antimicrobial therapy should be started promptly following thorough sampling and microbiological analysis. Empirical antibiotic treatment should target the most common causative organisms, including coagulase-negative staphylococci, *S. aureus* (or MRSA in high-prevalence settings), and potentially Gram-negative and anaerobic bacteria. Once microbiological culture results are obtained, targeted therapy should be initiated without delay [6, 8]. Linezolid is highly recommended due to its superior tissue penetration capabilities. In contrast, vancomycin is associated with poor tissue penetration, renal side effects, and limited efficacy against methicillin-resistant *Staphylococcus aureus* [51].

12 Wound Exploration

Early exploration of wounds with the patient under general anesthesia involves complete reopening of the sternotomy wound. All wires are removed, and cultures are taken to check for sepsis. If sepsis is present, the sternal edges are debrided until healthy bone with brisk bleeding margins is exposed. If the bone is necrotic, soft, and oozing pus, the entire sternum may need to be removed. Debridement is typically followed by packing with wet dressings and delayed closure at least 48 hours after the initial procedure.

Immediate wound closure using muscle flaps is crucial. Maintaining sternal stability during surgery is also important, and transverse fixation with titanium plates may be necessary. The pectoralis major flap is the preferred choice, followed by the rectus abdominis. The omentum and latissimus dorsi are also options, with the omentum being particularly useful due to its ability to conform to deep wound recesses. Drains are typically placed in both the muscle donor sites and the mediastinum for all patients [48, 49]. To assist in flap selection, Nahai et al. recommended pectoralis major muscle flap for defects in the upper half of the sternum, and the combined pectoralis major and rectus abdominis bi-pedicled muscle flaps for defects in the lower half and the whole sternum [52]. The timing of the reconstruction using muscle flaps is still debatable. Primary flap reconstruction is recommended by most scholars. For DSWI patients who cannot be treated with initial radical debridement, open and dressing are more important. Secondary tissue flap reconstruction should be conducted later [53].

The primary objectives of DSWI treatment are to control the infection through wound debridement and drainage including the removal of all infected tissues, dead bone and steel wire or sutures. After debridement, the muscle flap is used to close the infected area and obliterate the dead space. Drainage catheter tubes are inserted into infected areas, including the mediastinal cavity, muscle flap and dissected subcutaneous chest wall area. It is essential to conduct multiple bacterial cultures of wound secretions, sputum, and other relevant samples in DSWI patients upon admission, even if they do not exhibit clear symptoms of infection. This proactive approach allows for early detection and targeted treatment of any potential infections, ultimately improving patient outcomes [50].

13 Wound Reconstruction

In cases of DSWI with mediastinal infection and sternal instability, the common practice is to use either greater omentum transplantation or myocutaneous flap closure. Greater omentum is known for its ability to limit inflammation and prevent infection. It is rich in epidermal growth factor (EGF), which promotes epithelial synthesis protein, stimulates epithelial proliferation and migration, and is rich in vascular endothelial growth factor (VEGF) to aid in the reconstruction of blood supply in ischemic tissues. Compared to traditional debridement and closed drainage, muscle or omental flap reconstruction has shown lower complication rates and mortality rates of 22% and 0%, respectively, while the latter has complication and mortality rates of 92% and 33%, respectively [76].

Studies have indicated that in cases of wound infection with drug-resistant bacteria, greater omentum transplantation is preferred over muscle flaps [77]. Complications of omental transplantation may include epigastric hernia, bleeding, necrosis, massive exudation, and peritoneal cavity pollution [78].

The unilateral or bilateral pectoralis major myocutaneous flap is the most used method for reconstruction. According to Liu et al., this type of flap effectively fills residual cavities in cases of deep sternal wound infections (DSWI) [79]. Greig et al. also recommend the pectoralis major myocutaneous flap for closing severe upper sternal defects with more than 50% bone loss. In cases where the lower part of the sternum or the entire sternal space needs to be filled, options include the pedicled rectus abdominis, latissimus dorsi, or greater omentum. However, the rectus abdominis flap is near the wound and can be affected by inflammation for an extended period. Additionally, the internal thoracic artery may have been damaged during cardiac surgery, impacting the blood supply to the flaps [80]. Compared to the pectoralis major and rectus abdominis flaps, the latissimus dorsi flap is further away from potential infections, reducing the risk of local inflammatory invasion. It also has a rich blood supply and strong anti-infective properties, making it a favorable option for reconstruction [81].

14 Wound Care Management

14.1 Silver Dressings

An emerging trend in postoperative wound care involves the use of silver dressings to take advantage of the natural antibacterial properties of silver. Silver has a long history of success in coating medical devices and treating chronic wounds and burns. Recent studies have shown promising results in using silver dressings to prevent SSI [54–61]. Research has found that silver-impregnated surgical dressings applied to sternotomy wounds can significantly reduce the incidence of mediastinitis [62]. The interest in silver dressings in cardiac surgery was sparked by a study that showed a decrease in surgical wound infections to zero when silver dressings were used compared to traditional gauze in adult cardiac patients. Furthermore, another study demonstrated that adding silver dressings to patients with mediastinitis that did not respond to wound vacuum-assisted closure led to negative wound cultures. This highlights the potential benefits of incorporating silver dressings into postoperative wound care protocols [63, 64].

14.2 Negative Pressure Wound Therapy (NPWT)

NPWT is widely utilized for Surgical Wound Infections (SWI). It has been proven to enhance granulation tissue growth, increase wound drainage, and expedite cavity closure. In comparison to traditional mediastinal tube drainage post-debridement, NPWT offers superior treatment efficiency, decreased patient discomfort, and sustained debridement-like effects. NPWT operates by inducing a venous gradient hydrostatic pressure difference, facilitating fluid flow, reducing local osmotic active molecules, minimizing tissue edema, preventing microcirculation damage, preserving tissue perfusion, decreasing residual flushing fluid and inflammatory exudation, and notably alleviating patient pain. Additionally, NPWT stabilizes the sternum halves, leading to a shortened rehabilitation period [65–67].

NPWT not only minimizes patient discomfort but also maintains a continuous "debridement-like" effect. This innovative approach induces a venous gradient hydrostatic pressure difference, facilitating fluid flow and effectively reducing the presence of local osmotic active molecules. By decreasing tissue edema and minimizing microcirculation damage, NPWT ensures adequate tissue perfusion while also reducing residual flushing fluid and inflammatory exudation. Additionally, NPWT stabilizes the sternum halves, leading to a significant reduction in patient pain and a shortened rehabilitation period. NPWT helps remove fluid material, promote the formation of granulation tissue, assist in wound edge approximation, and promote the healing process. Negative Pressure Wound Therapy (NPWT) has been shown to significantly enhance patient health outcomes and provide economic benefits [68]. Applying continuous or intermittent negative pressure to a wound causes arteriolar dilatation, which in turn enhances wound perfusion and promotes the proliferation of granulation tissue [69].

NPWT should be initiated whenever possible in patients who are anticipated to have delayed sternal closure. To prevent tissue erosion and potentially fatal hemorrhage, it is crucial to utilize a dressing barrier between the sponge and the heart and great vessels when employing NPWT. This barrier serves as a protective layer, reducing the risk of complications and ensuring the safety of the patient during treatment [37, 53]. Several recent studies, meta-analyses, and systematic reviews have validated the efficacy of NPWT in DSWI either as a single-line therapy, or as a "bridge" prior to final surgical closure [7].

NPWT has shown success in treating MRSA mediastinitis and as a temporary treatment before secondary closure in mediastinitis caused by Candida [70]. Various studies have examined factors that may indicate NPWT failure. Gdalevitch and colleagues discovered that positive wound cultures, a wound depth of about 4 cm, and significant bony exposure and sternal instability are key predictors of NPWT failure [71]. The risk of secondary infection, the emergence of drug-resistant microorganisms, or erosion of vital structures like the right ventricle, large vessels, and bypass grafts leading to fatal bleeding can greatly impact the long-term healing outcomes of NPWT [20].

Gaudreau and team suggested that prolonged NPWT application could lead to chronic infection due to changes in bacterial species and increased growth of pathogens like *Staphylococcus aureus* [72].

The PrevenaTM Incision Management System, developed by Kinetic Concepts Inc. in San Antonio, TX, United States, is a cutting-edge surgical incision management system. This system utilizes a single-use Negative Pressure Wound Therapy (NPWT) to deliver a negative pressure ranging from 75 to 125 mmHg (10–16.7 KPa). The primary functions of this system include holding the incision edges together, reducing lateral tension and edema, stimulating perfusion, and providing protection to the surgical site against external infectious sources [73].

NPWT significantly enhances the healing process of SSWI compared to its limited effectiveness for DSWI accompanied by osteomyelitis or mediastinal infection. Combining NPWT with other treatments has been proven to yield more favorable outcomes. In a retrospective analysis conducted by Hao et al., 62 cases of DSWI with sternal osteomyelitis were examined. The study compared the sinus tract sealing time and wound healing time of patients treated with NPWT alone versus those treated with Platelet-Rich Plasma (PRP) in combination with NPWT. The results showed that the combination of PRP and NPWT had a significant positive impact on patients with DSWI and sternal osteomyelitis, leading to shorter sinus tract sealing time, faster wound healing, and a reduced need for secondary repair surgery.

Literature also suggests that NPWT alone may not be as effective in treating fungal infections, resulting in longer treatment times and a higher likelihood of reoperations. Therefore, it is important to consider alternative treatment options for patients with these specific conditions [74, 75].

Platelet-rich plasma (PRP) is a type of autologous plasma that contains high concentrations of platelets. This plasma can combat infections by releasing inflammatory inhibitory factors. Additionally, PRP can help alleviate surgical pain and neuropathic pain by regulating the body's inflammatory response, promoting regeneration, and restoring tissue innervation at the local level [82, 83].

Platelet-rich plasma (PRP) plays a crucial role in the entire tissue repair process, which includes hemostasis, inflammation, proliferation, and remodeling. Platelets are rich in α granules and high-density granules that secrete a variety of bioactive proteins. These proteins help regulate the migration and proliferation of keratinocytes, fibroblasts, and endothelial cells, promote angiogenesis, collagen synthesis, and epithelization, ultimately accelerating wound healing. In a study by Bielecki et al., it was found that PRP has an inhibitory effect on common bacteria such as *Staphylococcus aureus* and *Escherichia coli*, which are often present in surgical wound infections. This highlights the potential of PRP in preventing and treating infections in surgical wounds [84].

The positive impact of *platelet gel (PG)* on wound healing has been extensively documented in the literature. This treatment has the potential to decrease the occurrence of surgical site infections (SSI) [85, 86].

Antibiotic-loaded bone cement (ALBC) has been proven to have a therapeutic effect on osteomyelitis. Initially reported by Klemm, ALBC not only provides excellent mechanical support but also exhibits antibacterial properties. This innovative treatment has become widely utilized in the management of open fractures, osteomyelitis, and infections related to prostheses or foreign bodies [87, 88]. ALBC offers the advantage of being able to conform to the shape of the wound defects, ensuring complete filling of the residual cavity without creating dead space. Furthermore, it can be customized by incorporating various antibiotics based on the results of bacterial culture and drug sensitivity tests. This tailored approach not only provides mechanical support but also delivers targeted antibacterial action directly to the affected area.

Hyperbaric oxygen therapy (HBO2) has emerged as a promising treatment option for chronic and refractory wounds in recent years. This innovative therapy offers a range of benefits, including local anti-inflammatory effects, downregulation of cell adhesion molecules, reduction of leukocyte impact on endothelium, inhibition of anaerobic bacteria growth, promotion of angiogenesis, decreased edema, and enhanced collagen production [89]. A study conducted by Rados et al. assessed the efficacy and safety of HBO2 in patients with deep sternal wound infections (DSWI). The results were impressive, with an 80% success rate and no reported complications. This study highlights the potential of HBO2 as a valuable alternative for treating recurrent refractory DSWI cases [90].

15 Patient and Family Education on Incision Care

Proper care of the incision is crucial for optimal healing and to reduce the risk of infection. It is essential for patients to adhere to the following guidelines to ensure their incision heals satisfactorily, promotes successful recovery, and minimizes complications.

1. Daily Shower: Patients should shower daily using soap and water to keep the incision clean and free from bacteria.
2. Daily Inspection: It is imperative to inspect the incision daily using a mirror. Look for any signs of redness, irritation, swelling, tenderness, or unusual drainage. If any of these symptoms are present, contact the surgeon or the surgeon on call immediately. Patients should be able to recognize and list the signs and symptoms of infection for early detection and prompt medical attention if needed.
3. Dressing: A dressing is necessary only if there is drainage from the incision. If there is no drainage, a dressing is not required. Any dressings applied during the hospital stay should be removed the day after returning home to allow for better inspection of the incision and to promote healing.
4. Lifestyle Modifications: Patients should make necessary lifestyle changes to reduce risk factors that may hinder wound healing. This may include quitting smoking, maintaining a healthy diet, and managing chronic conditions.

References

1. Julian OC, Lopez-Belio M, Dye WS, Javid H, Grove WJ. The median sternal incision in intracardiac surgery with extracorporeal circulation: a general evaluation of its use in heart surgery. Surgery. 1957;42:753–61.
2. Jurkiewicz MJ, Arnold PG. The omentum: an account of its use in the reconstruction of the chest wall. Ann Surg. 1977;185(5):548–54. https://doi.org/10.1097/00000658-197705000-00007.
3. Edwards JR, Peterson KD, Mu Y, et al. National Healthcare Safety Network (NHSN) report: data summary for 2006 through 2008, issued December 2009. Am J Infect Control. 2009;37(10):783–805.
4. Jonkers D, Elenbaas T, Terporten P, Nieman F, Stobberingh E. Prevalence of 90-days postoperative wound infections after cardiac surgery. Eur J Cardiothorac Surg. 2003;23(1):97–102. https://doi.org/10.1016/s1010-7940(02)00662-0.
5. Naser N, Hadziomerovic N. Sudden cardiac deaths. IJBH. 2018;6(2):110–9. https://doi.org/10.5455/ijbh.2018.6.110-119.
6. Kotnis A, Mazur P, Olechowska A, Stanisz A, Bulanda M, Undas A. Sternal wound infections following cardiac surgery and their management: a single-centre study from the years 2016–2017. Kardiochir Torakochir Pol. 2018;15(2):79–85. https://doi.org/10.5114/kitp.2018.76472.
7. Cotogni P, Barbero C, Rinaldi M. Deep sternal wound infection after cardiac surgery: evidences and controversies. World J Crit Care Med. 2015;4(4):265–73. https://doi.org/10.5492/wjccm.v4.i4.265.
8. Banjanovic B, Karabdic IH, Straus S, Berberovic BH, MuhamedDjedovic NG. Deep sternal wound infection after open-heart cardiac surgery and vacuum-assisted losure therapy: a single-center study. Med Arch. 2022;76(4):273–7.
9. Mangram AJ, Horan TC, Pearson ML, Silver LC, Jarvis WR, Guideline for Prevention of Surgical Site Infection. Centers for Disease Control and Prevention (CDC) Hospital Infection Control Practices Advisory Committee. Am J Infect Control. 1999;27:97–132; quiz 133–134; discussion 96. PMID: 10196487. https://doi.org/10.1016/S0196-6553(99)70088-X.
10. Filsoufi F, Castillo JG, Rahmanian PB, Broumand SR, Silvay G, Carpentier A, Adams DH. Epidemiology of deep sternal wound infection in cardiac surgery. J Cardiothorac Vasc Anesth. 2009;23:488–94. PMID: 19376733. https://doi.org/10.1053/j.jvca.2009.02.007.

11. Braxton JH, Marrin CA, McGrath PD, Morton JR, Norotsky M, Charlesworth DC, Lahey SJ, Clough R, Ross CS, Olmstead EM, O'Connor GT. 10-year follow-up of patients with and without mediastinitis. Semin Thorac Cardiovasc Surg. 2004;16:70–6. PMID: 15366690.
12. Pairolero PC, Arnold PG. Management of recalcitrant median sternotomy wounds. J Thorac Cardiovasc Surg. 1984;88(3):357–64. Epub 1984/09/01.
13. Mujanovic E, Bergsland J, Jahic M, Djedovic S, Behrem A, Stanimirovic-Mujanovic S, et al. Bloodless off pump coronary artery bypass grafting, treatment of choice for Jehova's witness patients. Med Arch. 2012;66(2):140–2. https://doi.org/10.5455/medarh.2012.66.140-142.
14. Bergsland J. Development of cardiac services in Bosnia and Herzegovina - resource utilization and quality assurance: a perspective. Int J Biomedi Healthcare. 2021;9(4):288–93. https://doi.org/10.5455/ijbh.2021.9.288-293.
15. Cozza V, Pepe G, Cintoni M, De Maio F, Tropeano G, Mag-alini S, et al. Vacuum-Assisted Closure (VAC) systems and microbiological isolation of infected wounds. World J Emerg Surg. 2018;13:53. https://doi.org/10.1186/s13017-018-0216-z.
16. Kaye AE, Kaye AJ, Pahk B, McKenna ML, Low DW. Sternal wound reconstruction: management in different cardiac populations. Ann Plast Surg. 2010;64(5):658–66. Epub 2010/04/17.
17. Wang C, Zhang J, Liu Z. Vacuum-assisted closure therapy combined with bi-pectoral muscle ap for the treatment of deep sternal wound infections. Int Wound J. 2020;17:332–8. https://doi.org/10.1111/iwj.13277.
18. Baldassarro VA, Lorenzini L, Giuliani A, Cescatti M, Alastra G, Pannella M, et al. Molecular mechanisms of skin wound healing in non-diabetic and diabetic mice in excision and pressure experimental wounds. Cell Tissue Res. 2022;388(3):595–613. Pubmed Central PMCID: PMC9110453. Epub 2022/04/08.
19. Nikitina OV, Chainikova IN, Skachkova MA, Barsukova SV. Features of immunity in tobacco smoking among adolescents. Gig Sanit. 2012;3:59–61. Epub 2012/10/24.
20. Alebrahim K, Al-Ebrahim E. Prevention. Classification and management review of deep sternal wound infection. Heart Surg Forum. 2020;23(5):E652–E7. Epub 2020/09/30.
21. Raanani E, Spiegelstein D, Sternik L, Preisman S, Moshkovitz Y, Smolinsky AK, et al. Quality of mitral valve repair: median sternotomy versus port-access approach. J Thorac Cardiovasc Surg. 2010;140(1):86–90. Epub 2009/12/09.
22. Vitartaite M, Vaiciulyte D, Vencloviene J, Sirvinskas E, Bukauskiene R, Jakuska P, et al. Risk factors associated with an increased risk of deep sternal wound infections in patients after coronary artery bypass grafting and heart defect surgery. Heart Surg Forum. 2021;24(4):E741–E5. Epub 2021/09/03.
23. Saso S, James D, Vecht JA, Kidher E, Kokotsakis J, Malinovski V, Rao C, Darzi A, Anderson JR, Athanasiou T. Effect of skeletonization of the internal thoracic artery for coronary revascularization on the incidence of sternal wound infection. Ann Thorac Surg. 2010;89:661–70. PMID: 20103378. https://doi.org/10.1016/j.athoracsur.2009.08.018.
24. Culver DH, Horan TC, Gaynes RP, Martone WJ, Jarvis WR, Emori TG, Banerjee SN, Edwards JR, Tolson JS, Henderson TS, et al. Surgical wound infection rates by wound class, operative procedure, and patient risk index. National Nosocomial Infections Surveillance System. Am J Med. 1991;91(3B):152S–7S. https://doi.org/10.1016/0002-9343(91)90361-z.
25. Song Y, Chu W, Sun J, Zhu H, Liu X, Yul H. Review on risk factors, classification, and treatment of stenal woind infection. J Cardiothorac Surg. 2003;18:184. https://doi.org/10.1186/s13019-023-2228-y.
26. FZ RFZ, TH LN, WJ QF. 18F-FDG PET/CT guided management of infective costal chondritis after cardiac surgery. Chin J Aesthetic Med. 2018;27(2):28.
27. Irmler IM, Opfermann T, Gebhardt P, Gajda M, Brauer R, Saluz HP, et al. In vivo molecular imaging of experimental joint in ammation by combined (18) F-FDG positron emission tomography and computed tomography. Arthritis Res Ther. 2010;12(6):R203. Pubmed Central PMCID: PMC3046507. Epub 2010/11/05.
28. Gur E, Stern D, Weiss J, Herman O, Wertheym E, Cohen M, et al. Clinical-radio- logical evaluation of poststernotomy wound infection. Plast Reconstr Surg. 1998;101(2):348–55. Epub 1998/02/14.

29. Sjögren J, Malmsjö M, Gustafsson R, Ingemansson R. Post- sternotomy mediastinitis: a review of conventional surgical treatments, vacuum-assisted closure therapy and presentation of the Lund University Hospital mediastinitis algorithm. Eur J Cardiothorac Surg. 2006;30:898–905. PMID: 17056269. https://doi.org/10.1016/j.jects.2006.09.020.
30. National Nosocomial Infections Surveillance System. National Nosocomial Infections Surveillance (NNIS) System Report, data summary from January 1992 through June 2004, issued October 2004. Am J Infect Control. 2004;32:470–85. PMID: 15573054. https://doi.org/10.1016/j.ajic.2004.10.001.
31. Goh SSC. Post-sternotomy mediastinitis in the modern era. J Card Surg. 2017;32(9):556–66. PMID: 28833518.
32. von Eckardstein AS, Lim CH, Dohmen PM, et al. A randomized trial of a skin sealant to reduce the risk of incision contamination in cardiac surgery. Ann Thorac Surg. 2011;92(2):632–7. PMID: 21704290.
33. Mossad SB, Serkey JM, Longworth DL, Cosgrove DM 3rd, Gordon SM. Coagulase-negative staphylococcal sternal wound infections after open heart operations. Ann Thorac Surg. 1997;63(2):395–401. PMID: 9033307.
34. Gårdlund B, Bitkover CY, Vaage J. Postoperative mediastinitis in cardiac surgery - microbiology and pathogenesis. Eur J Cardiothorac Surg. 2002;21(5):825–30. PMID: 12062270.
35. Losanoff JE, Richman BW, Jones JW. Disruption and infection of median sternotomy: a comprehensive review. Eur J Cardiothorac Surg. 2002;21(5):831–9. PMID: 12062271.
36. Majid FM, Buba FM, Barry M, Alsharani F, Alfawzan F. Incidence, types and outcomes of sternal wound infections after cardiac surgery in Saudi Arabia. Saudi Med J. 2020;41(2):177–82. https://doi.org/10.15537/smj.2020.2.24843.
37. Lazar HL, Salm TV, Engelman R, Orgill D, Gordon S. Prevention, and management of sternal wound infections. J Thorac Cardiovasc Surg. 2016;152(4):962–72. https://doi.org/10.1016/j.jtcvs.2016.01.060. Epub 2016 Aug 8. PMID: 27555340.
38. Engelman R, Shahian D, Shemin R, Guy TS, Bratzler D, Edwards F, Jacobs M, Fernando H, Bridges C, Workforce on Evidence-Based Medicine, Society of Thoracic Surgeons. The Society of Thoracic Surgeons practice guideline series: antibiotic prophylaxis in cardiac surgery, part II: antibiotic choice. Ann Thorac Surg. 2007;83:1569–76. PMID: 17383396. https://doi.org/10.1016/j.athoracsur.2006.09.046.
39. Galbraith U, Schilling J, von Segesser LK, Carrel T, Turina M, Geroulanos S. Antibiotic prophylaxis in cardiovascular surgery: a prospective randomized comparative trial of one day cefazolin versus single dose cefuroxime. Drugs Exp Clin Res. 1993;19:229–34. PMID: 8174496.
40. Townsend TR, Reitz BA, Bilker WB, Bartlett JG. Clinical trial of cefamandole, cefazolin, and cefuroxime for antibiotic prophylaxis in cardiac operations. J Thorac Cardiovasc Surg. 1993;106:664–70. PMID: 8412261.
41. Cotogni P, Passera R, Barbero C, Gariboldi A, Moscato D, Izzo G, Rinaldi M. Intraoperative vancomycin pharmacokinetics in cardiac surgery with or without cardiopulmonary bypass. Ann Pharmacother. 2013;47:455–63. PMID: 23512663. https://doi.org/10.1345/aph.1R669.
42. Bolon MK, Morlote M, Weber SG, Koplan B, Carmeli Y, Wright SB. Glycopeptides are no more effective than beta-lactam agents for prevention of surgical site infection after cardiac surgery: a meta-analysis. Clin Infect Dis. 2004;38(10):1357–63. https://doi.org/10.1086/383318. Epub 2004 Apr 21. PMID: 15156470.
43. Caffarelli AD, Holden JP, Baron EJ, Lemmens HJ, D'Souza H, Yau V, Olcott C, Reitz BA, Miller DC, van der Starre PJ. Plasma cefazolin levels during cardiovascular surgery: effects of cardiopulmonary bypass and profound hypothermic circulatory arrest. J Thorac Cardiovasc Surg. 2006;131:1338–43. PMID: 16733167. https://doi.org/10.1016/j.jtcvs.2005.11.047.
44. Edwards FH, Engelman RM, Houck P, Shahian DM, Bridges CR. The society of thoracic surgeons practice guideline series: antibiotic prophylaxis in cardiac surgery, part I: duration. Ann Thorac Surg. 2006;81:397–404. PMID: 16368422. https://doi.org/10.1016/j.athoracsur.2005.06.034.

45. Bratzler DW, Hunt DR. The surgical infection prevention and surgical care improvement projects: national initiatives to improve outcomes for patients having surgery. Clin Infect Dis. 2006;43:322–30. PMID: 16804848. https://doi.org/10.1086/505220.
46. Ma JG, An JX. Deep sternal wound infection after cardiac surgery: a comparison of three different wound infection types and an analysis of antibiotic resistance. J Thorac Dis. 2018;10(1):377–87. https://doi.org/10.21037/jtd.2017.12.109. PMID: 29600070; PMCID: PMC5863177.
47. Pairolero PC, Arnold PG. Management of infected median sternotomy wounds. Ann Thorac Surg. 1986;42(1):1–2. https://doi.org/10.1016/s0003-4975(10)61822-x. PMID: 3729602.
48. Jones G, Jurkiewicz MJ, Bostwick J, Wood R, Bried JT, Culbertson J, Howell R, Eaves F, Carlson G, Nahai F. Management of the infected median sternotomy wound with muscle flaps. The Emory 20-year experience. Ann Surg. 1997;225(6):766–76; discussion 776–8. PMID: 9230817; PMCID: PMC1190886. https://doi.org/10.1097/00000658-199706000-00014.
49. Ridderstolpe L, Gill H, Granfeldt H, Ahlfeldt H, Rutberg H. Superficial and deep sternal wound complications: incidence, risk factors and mortality. Eur J Cardiothorac Surg. 2001;20(6):1168–75. https://doi.org/10.1016/s1010-7940(01)00991-5. PMID: 11717023.
50. Elassal AA, Al-Ebrahim KE, Al-Radi OO, Jabbad HH, Eldib OS. Sternal wound complications: objective reclassification and surgical reconsideration. Heart Surg Forum. 2020;23(1):E076–E80. PubMed PMID: 32118548. Epub 2020/03/03.
51. Reineke S, Carrel TP, Eigenmann V, Gahl B, Fuehrer U, Seidl C, et al. Adding vancomycin to perioperative prophylaxis decreases deep sternal wound infections in high-risk cardiac surgery patients. Eur J Cardiothorac Surg. 2018;53(2):428–34. PubMed PMID: 29045740. Epub 2017/10/19.
52. Nahai F, Rand RP, Hester TR, Bostwick J 3rd, Jurkiewicz MJ. Primary treatment of the infected sternotomy wound with muscle flaps: a review of 211 consecutive cases. Plast Reconstr Surg. 1989;84:434e441.
53. Shi YD, Qi FZ, Zhang Y. Treatment of sternal wound infections after open-heart surgery. Asian J Surg. 2014;37(1):24–9. https://doi.org/10.1016/j.asjsur.2013.07.006. Epub 2013 Aug 22. PMID: 23972506.
54. Krieger BR, Davis DM, Sanchez JE, et al. The use of silver nylon in preventing surgical site infections following colon and rectal surgery. Dis Colon Rectum. 2011;54(8):1014–9. PMID: 21730792.
55. Epstein NE. Do silver-impregnated dressings limit infections after lumbar laminectomy with instrumented fusion? Surg Neurol. 2007;68(5):483–5. PMID: 17961738.
56. Zegelman M, Guenther G, Waliszewski M, et al. Results from the international silver graft registry for high-risk patients treated with a metallic silver impregnated vascular graft. Vascular. 2013;21(3):137–47. PMID: 23508393.
57. Ogbemudia AO, Bafor A, Edomwonyi E, Enemudo R. Prevalence of pin tract infection: the role of combined silver sulphadiazine and chlorhexidine dressing. Niger J Clin Pract. 2010;13(3):268–71. PMID: 20857782.
58. Nherera L, Trueman P, Roberts C, Berg L. Silver delivery approaches in the management of partial thickness burns: a systematic review and indirect treatment comparison. Wound Repair Regen. 2017;25(4):707–21. PMID: 28742235.
59. Moir J, Serra MP. The use of silver nitrate in wound management. Ann Ital Chir. 2012;83(1):45–8. PMID: 22352216.
60. Storm-Versloot MN, Vos CG, Ubbink DT, Vermeulen H. Topical silver for preventing wound infection. Cochrane Database Syst Rev. 2010;3:CD006478. PMID: 20238345.
61. Siah CJ, Yatim J. Efficacy of a total occlusive ionic silver-containing dressing combination in decreasing risk of surgical site infection: an RCT. J Wound Care. 2011;20(12):561–8. PMID: 22240882.
62. Staveski S, Abrajano C, Casazza M, et al. Silver-impregnated dressings for sternotomy incisions to prevent surgical site infections in children. Am J Crit Care. 2016;25(5):402–8. PMID: 27587419.

63. Huckfeldt R, Redmond C, Mikkelson D, Finley PJ, Lowe C, Robertson J. A clinical trial to investigate the effect of silver nylon dressings on mediastinitis rates in postoperative cardiac sternotomy incisions. Ostomy Wound Manage. 2008;54(10):36–41. PMID: 18927482.
64. Totaro P, Rambaldini M. Efficacy of antimicrobial activity of slow-release silver nanoparticles dressing in post-cardiac surgery mediastinitis. Interact Cardiovasc Thorac Surg. 2009;8(1):153–4. PMID: 18948308.
65. Drossos G, Ampatzidou F, Baddour A, Madesis A, Karaiskos T. The impact of deep sternal wound infections treated by negative pressure on early, 1 year and late mortality: a longitudinal case-control study. J Card Surg. 2019;34(12):1550–5. PubMed PMID: 31654592. Epub 2019/10/28.
66. Gatti G, Benussi B, Brunetti D, Ceschia A, Porcari A, Biondi F, et al. The fate of patients having deep sternal infection after bilateral internal thoracic artery grafting in the negative pressure wound therapy era. Int J Cardiol. 2018;269:67–74. PubMed PMID: 30049494. Epub 2018/07/28.
67. Gatti G, Ledwon M, Gazdag L, Cuomo F, Pappalardo A, Fischlein T, et al. Management of closed sternal incision after bilateral internal thoracic artery grafting with a single-use negative pressure system. Updat Surg. 2018;70(4):545–52. PubMed PMID: 29460174. Epub 2018/02/21.
68. Yusuf E, Chan M, Renz N, Trampuz A. Current perspectives on diagnosis and management of sternal wound infections. Infect Drug Resist. 2018;11:961–8. https://doi.org/10.2147/IDR.S130172.
69. Ennker IC, Pietrowski D, Vöhringer L, Kojcici B, Albert A, Vogt PM, Ennker J. Surgical debridement, vacuum therapy and pectoralis plasty in poststernotomy mediastinitis. J Plast Reconstr Aesthet Surg. 2009;62:1479–83. PMID: 18996074. https://doi.org/10.1016/j.bjps.2008.05.017.
70. Osada H, Nakajima H, Morishima M, Su T. Candidal mediastinitis successfully treated using vacuum-assisted closure following open- heart surgery. Interact Cardiovasc Thorac Surg. 2012;14:872–4. PMID: 22422875. https://doi.org/10.1093/icvts/ivs084.
71. Gdalevitch P, Afilalo J, Lee C. Predictors of vacuum-assisted closure failure of sternotomy wounds. J Plast Reconstr Aesthet Surg. 2010;63:180–3. PMID: 19028156. https://doi.org/10.1016/j.bjps.2008.08.020.
72. Gaudreau G, Costache V, Houde C, Cloutier D, Montalin L, Voisine P, Baillot R. Recurrent sternal infection following treatment with negative pressure wound therapy and titanium transverse plate fixation. Eur J Cardiothorac Surg. 2010;37:888–92. PMID: 19775906. https://doi.org/10.1016/j.ejcts.2009.07.043.
73. Dohmen PM, Misfeld M, Borger MA, Mohr FW. Closed incision management with negative pressure wound therapy. Expert Rev Med Devices. 2014;11:395–402. PMID: 24754343. https://doi.org/10.1586/17434440.2014.911081.
74. Hao D, Feng G, Li T, Chu W, Chen Z, Li S, et al. Curative effects of platelet- rich plasma combined with negative-pressure wound therapy on sternal osteomyelitis and sinus tract after thoracotomy. Zhonghua Shao Shang Za Zhi. 2016;32(6):331–5. PubMed PMID: 27321486. Epub 2016/06/21.
75. Hamalainen E, Laurikka J, Huhtala H, Jarvinen O. Vacuum assistance therapy as compared to early reconstructive treatment in deep sternal wound infection. Scand J Surg. 2021;110(2):248–53. PubMed PMID: 33327852. Pubmed Central PMCID: PMC8258712. Epub 2020/12/18.
76. Brandt C, Alvarez JM. First-line treatment of deep sternal infection by a plastic surgical approach: superior results compared with conventional cardiac surgical orthodoxy. Plast Reconstr Surg. 2002;109(7):2231–7. PubMed PMID: 12045542 Epub 2001/10/09.
77. Botianu PVH. Current indications for the intrathoracic transposition of the omentum. J Cardiothorac Surg. 2019;14(1):103. PubMed PMID: 31182112. Pubmed Central PMCID: PMC6558767. Epub 2019/06/12.
78. Tewarie L, Moza AK, Khattab MA, Autschbach R, Zayat R. Effective combination of different surgical strategies for deep sternal wound infection and mediastinitis. Ann Thorac

Cardiovasc Surg. 2019;25(2):102–10. PubMed PMID: 30404980. Pubmed Central PMCID: PMC6477456. Epub 2018/11/09.
79. Jifu LIU, Yongshun GAO, Baocheng LI, Xiaobin XU, Shuo HUANG. New technique of pectoral muscle ap reconstruction for 23 patients with deep sernal wound infections. Chin J Clin Thorac Cardiovasc Surg. 2018;12:321–4. Article in Chinese.
80. Greig AV, Geh JL, Khanduja V, Shibu M. Choice of ap for the management of deep sternal wound infection–an anatomical classi cation. J Plast Reconstr Aesthet Surg. 2007;60(4):372–8. PubMed PMID: 17349591. Epub 2007/03/14.
81. Deng Guosan KBCY, Shifeng K, Guangxiang H, Chengli Z, Jian D, Jihong L, Wenbin X. Application of latissimus dorsi myocutaneous ap in repair of sternal incision infection and rupture after coronary artery bypass grafting. Chin J Surg. 2005;43(3):195.
82. Sethi D, Martin KE, Shrotriya S, Brown BL. Systematic literature review evaluating evidence and mechanisms of action for platelet-rich plasma as an antibacterial agent. J Cardiothorac Surg. 2021;16(1):277. PubMed PMID: 34583720. Pubmed Central PMCID: PMC8480088. Epub 2021/09/30.
83. Patel AN, Selzman CH, Kumpati GS, McKellar SH, Bull DA. Evaluation of autologous platelet rich plasma for cardiac surgery: outcome analysis of 2000 patients. J Cardiothorac Surg. 2016;11(1):62. https://doi.org/10.1186/s13019-016-0452-9. PMID: 27068030; PMCID: PMC4828785.
84. Yao D, Feng G, Zhao F, Hao D. Effects of platelet-rich plasma on the healing of sternal wounds: a meta-analysis. Wound Repair Regen. 2021;29(1):153–67. PubMed PMID: 33128501. Epub 2020/11/01.
85. Englert SJ, Estep TH, Ellis-Stoll CC. Autologous platelet gel applications during cardiovascular surgery: effect on wound healing. J Extra Corpor Technol. 2005;37(2):148–52. PMID: 16117450; PMCID: PMC4682529.
86. Everts PA, Knape JT, Weibrich G, Schönberger JP, Hoffmann J, Overdevest EP, Box HA, van Zundert A. Platelet-rich plasma and platelet gel: a review. J Extra Corpor Technol. 2006;38(2):174–87. PMID: 16921694; PMCID: PMC4680757.
87. Klemm KW. Gentamicin-PMMA chains (Septopal chains) for the local antibiotic treatment of chronic osteomyelitis. Reconstr Surg Traumatol. 1988;20:11–35. PubMed PMID: 3399737. Epub 1988/01/01.
88. Jiang X, Bu F, Xu Y, Jing Z, Jiao G, Li M, et al. Antibiotic-loaded bone cement combined with vacuum sealing drainage to treat deep sternal wound infection following cardiac surgery: the rst case report. J Cardiothorac Surg. 2021;16(1):292. PubMed PMID: 34629078. Pubmed Central PMCID: PMC8504067. Epub 2021/10/12.
89. Fevrier A, Boursot C, Tannugi KC. Osteomyelitis and gentamicin-PMMA chains. Clin Nucl Med. 2022;47(11):e708–e9. PubMed PMID: 35961640. Epub 2022/08/13.
90. Litwinowicz R, Bryndza M, Chrapusta A, Kobielska E, Kapelak B, Grudzien G. Hyperbaric oxygen therapy as additional treatment in deep sternal wound infections—a single center's experience. Kardiochir Torakochirurgia Pol. 2016;13(3):198–202. PubMed PMID: 27785131. Pubmed Central PMCID: PMC5071585. Epub 2016/10/28.

Hematology Management After Cardiac Surgery: Postoperative Care

Noora Al-Hail, Malek Abusannuga, and Mahmoud Ibrahim Abdelmoati

Objective

1. To provide a comprehensive overview of hematologic changes associated with cardiac surgery
2. To elucidate the pathophysiology, prevalence, and clinical implication of hematologic complications such as anemia, coagulopathy, and thrombocytopenia
3. To highlight the role of diagnostic tools, including thromboelastography(TEG) and rotational thromboelastometry (ROTEM), in improving postoperative management.
4. To emphasize evidence-based management strategies for optimizing transfusion practice and reducing complication.

1 Introduction

As with many complex procedures, cardiovascular surgeries can significantly impact multiple systems throughout the body. One of the most significant complications is coagulopathy, which is a condition that may result in long hospitalization, reoperation, and sever bleeding. Such complications escalate health expenditure as

N. Al-Hail (✉)
Department of Otorhinolaryngology, Head and Neck Surgery (ENT), Hamad Medical Corporation, Doha, Qatar

Department of Medical Education, Hamad Medical Corporation, Doha, Qatar
e-mail: nalhail@hamad.qa

M. Abusannuga
Anaesthesia, ICU and Perioperative Medicine Department, Hamad Medical Corporation, Doha, Qatar

M. I. Abdelmoati
Royal College of Surgeons in Ireland Medical University of Bahrain, Manamah, Bahrain

E. Elmistekawy, N. A. Shallik (eds.), *Perioperative Care of Cardiac Surgery Patients*, https://doi.org/10.1007/978-3-032-09817-7_6

well as mortality. Thus, the appropriate and timely recognition and treatment of coagulopathy is very important in the patient's health outcome and recovery phase. Hence, it is important to understand the hematological alteration in the patient's blood post-cardiac surgery, including the pathopsychological mechanisms and clinical implications. To optimize the patient positive operative outcome, it is essential to implement evidence-based management strategies and integrate advance diagnostics like TEG and ROTEM. The overall goal is to effectively diagnose and manage patient's post-cardiac surgery.

2 Description of Common Hematologic Alterations and Anemia After Surgery

- *Cause of Anemia After Cardiac Surgery*:
  1. *Hemodilution*:
     Hemodilution is one of the common results of using high volumes of intravenous fluids in cardiac surgery. This causes a dilution of blood components such as red blood cells (RBCs), platelets, and plasma proteins, lowering the hematocrit level and resulting in acute anemia. Low hemoglobin levels then compromise blood's oxygen-carrying capacity to tissues. Hemodilution also exacerbates clotting disorders by diluting platelets and clotting factors, thus raising the risk of bleeding and transfusion[11].
  2. *Blood Loss*:
     Anemia in heart surgery patients is primarily due to intraoperative and postoperative blood loss. Intraoperative blood loss during cardiopulmonary bypass (CPB) treatments can range from 300 to 400 mL, which is primarily due to surgical bleeding and suctioning in the operating field. CPB circuits also retain a portion of the blood volume, leading to further RBC depletion. Postoperative blood loss, which might be increased at chest drainage, continues for hours or days following a surgical procedure, so it continues aggravating anemia postoperatively. Literature shows that both intra- and postoperative losses contribute towards low postoperative levels of hematocrit and hemoglobin. For instance, Nelson et al. [31] report that the average total RBC loss before and after CPB surgery is about 38%, which is a significant predictor of acute anemia.
  3. *Inadequate Erythropoiesis*:
     Systemic inflammation results from surgery, causing higher levels of pro-inflammatory cytokines like IL-6 and TNF-α. These cytokines suppress the generation of EPO in the kidneys. EPO is an important hormone that promotes the synthesis of RBCs in the bone marrow. Lowered levels of EPO, combined with the suppressive effects of inflammation on erythroid progenitor cells, slow the recovery of RBCs following blood loss during surgery. In addition, the inflammatory marker hepcidin, increased in this response, inhibits mobilization of iron, necessary for hemoglobin synthesis, which also hampers erythropoiesis. Researchers have indicated that

this inhibition may prolong postoperative anemia and increase the demands for blood transfusions, which are known to carry extra risks. Erythropoiesis-stimulating drugs and iron supplementation are currently being researched as potential measures.

4. *Hemolysis*:

   Mechanical damage and shear stress induced by CPB circuits are major contributors to anemia after heart surgery. As blood flows through the CPB system, it is exposed to strong shear stresses, turbulence, and contact with non-endothelial surfaces, leading to RBC rupture. RBC lysis results in the release of free hemoglobin into the plasma, which can exacerbate oxidative stress and inflammation. Based on the findings, the level of hemolysis is related to CPB duration and circuit design. In addition to that, the free hemoglobin produced in the process of hemolysis may combine with nitric oxide, leading to an impairment in vascular function and resulting in conditions such as vasoconstriction and thrombosis. This hemolytic process not only decreases the oxygen-carrying capacity of blood but worsens postoperative anemia as well.

- *Prevalence*:

  The prevalence of preoperative anemia is 15–54%. Nguyen et al. [32] showed that 15% of the patients included in their study that underwent elective heart surgery were reported to have anemia before their surgery, and they were reported to have received more transfusions. Literature shows that in 75–90% of patients getting cardiac surgery postoperative anemia is reported, which mainly occurs due to internal blood loss during operations, CPB-induced hemolysis, and a delayed erythropoietin response [24]. Surgery promotes a systemic inflammatory response that can further reduce erythropoiesis, therefore continuing anemia. Moderate to severe anemia following surgery has been linked to greater morbidity, longer hospital admissions, and higher fatality rates [23].

3 Coagulation Changes and Risk of Bleeding During Cardiac Surgery

Cardiac surgeries, especially those involving CPB, can cause significant alterations in hemostasis, leading to both hypercoagulability and an increased risk of bleeding. The key mechanisms and contributing factors include [1]:

- *Effects of Anesthesia*
  - *Hemodilution*: Volume expansion from anesthetic management exacerbates hemodilution; in addition to, infusion of crystalloids, colloids, or banked blood further dilutes clotting factors, platelets, and fibrinogen [35].
  - *Hypothermia*: Mild hypothermia employed during surgery impairs enzymatic activity in the coagulation cascade and alters platelet function [2].
- *Consumption of Coagulation Factors and Contact Activation*:

  - Cardiac significantly affects coagulation primarily by activating coagulation cascades and consuming clotting factors and platelets. During CPB, Blood interaction with non-endothelial surfaces of the bypass circuit initiates the intrinsic coagulation pathway through contact activation. Results in the activation of factor XII (Hageman factor), leading to a cascade of reactions leading to thrombin generation and fibrin formation [41]. Concurrently, the activation of these cascades consumes circulating clotting factors such as fibrinogen, prothrombin, and platelets, resulting in a coagulopathy state characterized by reduced clotting potential [47].
- *Platelet Dysfunction*:
  - Platelets can become dysfunctional due to shear stress, hypothermia during surgery, and contact with synthetic surfaces, which break membranes and decrease function [15]. Additionally, contact with the CPB circuit's synthetic surfaces causes platelet activation, which, while initially aiding clot formation, eventually depletes platelet reserves and diminishes their ability to form effective clots. This increased activation and aggregation causes thrombocytopenia and poor clot formation, increasing the risk of bleeding. The systemic inflammatory response and the use of anticoagulants, both of which inhibit platelet-mediated hemostasis, worsen CPB-induced platelet dysfunction [34].
- *Fibrinolysis*
  - Cardiac surgery increases fibrinolytic activity by activating plasminogen and blocking natural antifibrinolytic processes, causing an imbalance in fibrin breakdown and synthesis. Tissue plasminogen activator (tPA) is released in response to vascular endothelial stress, converting plasminogen to plasmin, the enzyme that degrades fibrin. Reduce antifibrinolytic drugs, including α2-antiplasmin and thrombin-activatable fibrinolysis inhibitor (TAFI), to enhance fibrinolytic activity. This hyperfibrinolytic state can result in increased bleeding due to rapid clot breakdown and decreased clot stability. Furthermore, mechanical and inflammatory stressors promote the release of pro-fibrinolytic mediators, raising the risk of bleeding [36, 39].
- *Thrombocytopenia*
  - Thrombocytopenia is a common hematological alteration after cardiac surgery resulting from multiple mechanisms. This includes the shear stress, activating and aggregating platelets, which leads to their consumption and reduction in circulating levels. Concurrently, the large fluid volumes used during surgery and subsequent blood transfusions dilute the platelet concentration, compounding the drop in counts. Heparin-Induced Thrombocytopenia can trigger an immune-mediated drop in platelet count in 1–3% of patients. Effective management of thrombocytopenia post-surgery requires a multifactorial approach, including monitoring platelet counts, evaluating for HIT, and optimizing transfusion strategies [21, 22, 42].
  - Prevalence: Mild thrombocytopenia (platelets <150,000/μL) is common after CPB occurs in 90–100% of patients. Severe thrombocytopenia (<50,000/μL) occurs in 5–10% of cases.

- *Inflammation and Endothelial Dysfunction*
  - Cardiac surgery causes a systemic inflammatory response syndrome (SIRS), affecting endothelial function and coagulation mechanisms. SIRS starts when immunological pathways activate, releasing inflammatory cytokines such TNF-α and interleukins. These cytokines stimulate endothelial cells, contributing to coagulation cascade dysregulation [44]. The active endothelium becomes pro-thrombotic, increasing tissue factor expression and von Willebrand factor release, both of which are necessary for clot formation and platelet aggregation. Furthermore, endothelial injury exacerbates coagulopathy by disrupting the delicate balance of coagulation and fibrinolysis. It leads to profuse bleeding, thrombosis, and capillary leak syndrome.
- *Effects of Transfusion of Stored Blood*:
  - Storage changes the blood biochemically and structurally, such as a decrease in the level of 2,3-DPG. This reduces hemoglobin's ability to offload oxygen, which may exacerbate hypoxia in heart surgery patients recovering from the procedure [14]. The proinflammatory mediators and microparticles are accumulated during long-term storage, which worsens postoperative systemic inflammatory response syndrome (SIRS) with banked blood [50]. The immunomodulatory effect of blood transfusions has also been demonstrated; transfused plasma components and leukocytes can modulate the immunological response in the recipient and increase the chance of infection. In addition, transfused platelets may show abnormal aggregation, which could increase the chance of thrombotic complications such as pulmonary embolism or deep vein thrombosis. These risks are already high for patients undergoing cardiac surgery because of hypercoagulability and endothelial damage [50].
- *Preexisting and Perioperative Factors*
  - Patients with previous coagulopathies, such as liver disease or anticoagulant use, are more likely to experience complications.
  - Intraoperative heparin injection and protamine reversal may result in inadequate neutralization or rebound anticoagulation [7, 27].

4 Assessment and Monitoring in Postoperative Hematology Care

Effective hematological assessment and monitoring are essential in managing the postoperative course following cardiac surgery. Cardiac surgery induces significant changes in coagulation due to hemodilution, platelet dysfunction, fibrinolysis, and inflammation [17]. These measures enable timely detection and intervention for bleeding, coagulopathy, or thrombotic complications [13].

Laboratory Tests and Monitoring Protocols

1. *Complete Blood Count (CBC)*:
   - *Purpose*: Assesses hemoglobin, hematocrit, and white blood cell levels.
   - *Clinical Use*: Identifies anemia (common postoperatively due to blood loss or dilution), leukocytosis (infection or inflammation), and leukopenia (immunosuppression or specific conditions) [40].
2. *Coagulation Profile*:
   - *Tests*: Prothrombin Time (PT), Activated Partial Thromboplastin Time (aPTT), and International Normalized Ratio (INR).
   - *Purpose*: Evaluates intrinsic and extrinsic coagulation pathways.
   - *Clinical Use*: Identifies coagulopathy due to anticoagulant therapy, liver dysfunction, or factor deficiencies. PT/INR guides FFP or vitamin K administration, whereas prolonged aPTT can signal heparin use or factor deficiency.
3. *Platelet Count*:
   - *Purpose*: Detects thrombocytopenia, a frequent issue in cardiac surgery, often resulting from platelet activation and destruction.
   - *Clinical Use*: According to Warkentin et al. [48], decisions related to platelet transfusion ought to be guided at platelet counts below 50,000/μL along with hemorrhage or 100,000/μL in high-risk conditions.
4. *Fibrinogen Levels*:
   - *Purpose*: Monitors depletion of fibrinogen is a common factor seen in problems related to bleeding.
   - *Clinical Use*: Levels below 2 g/L indicate that fibrinogen must be concentrate or cryoprecipitate for the clot strength to improve.
5. *Viscoelastic Testing*:
   - *ROTEM (Rotational Thromboelastometry) and TEG (Thromboelastography)*:
     - Provides dynamic assessments of clot formation, firmness, and fibrinolysis.
     - Identifies particular deficits, such as hypofibrinogenemia or hyperfibrinolysis, for targeted therapy with fibrinogen concentrate or antifibrinolytics [8].
6. *D-dimer and Fibrinolysis Markers*:
   - *Purpose*: Monitors for excessive fibrinolysis or thrombotic states.
   - *Clinical Use*: Elevated D-dimer levels in conjunction with TEG/ROTEM findings may indicate hyperfibrinolysis or microthrombosis.

5 Interpretation of Results and Clinical Implications

1. *Anemia or Low Hematocrit*:
   - Red blood cell transfusion is necessary if symptomatic or below critical thresholds (<7–8 g/dL in stable patients or <10 g/dL in high-risk situations) [3].

2. *Coagulopathy*:
   - Coagulopathy can be managed by correcting extended PT/INR with vitamin K, fresh frozen plasma (FFP), or factor concentrates.
3. *Thrombocytopenia or Platelet Dysfunction*:
   - Platelet transfusion is recommended for counts <50,000/μL with bleeding or <100,000/μL in high-risk scenarios (American Society of Hematology 2018).
4. *Hyperfibrinolysis*:
   - Treated with antifibrinolytics such as tranexamic acid or aminocaproic acid, guided by ROTEM/TEG findings.

6 Management Strategies for Hematologic Issues in Cardiac Surgery Patients

Hematologic complications are common in patients undergoing cardiac surgery. The following strategies address key hematologic challenges postoperatively:

6.1 Management of Anemia Post-surgery

1. *Iron Supplementation and Erythropoiesis-Stimulating Agents (ESAs)*
   Postoperative anemia is often treated with iron supplementation and erythropoiesis-stimulating agents (ESAs). Intravenous iron is preferred for rapid replenishment of iron stores, especially in cases of functional iron deficiency where oral iron may be less effective [6]. ESAs, such as recombinant erythropoietin, are used to stimulate red blood cell production, particularly in patients at risk of developing severe anemia or with contraindications to transfusions. Evidence indicates that combining ESAs with iron supplementation significantly enhances erythropoiesis compared to either treatment alone, reducing transfusion requirements and improving recovery outcomes [10]. However, these interventions must be carefully tailored, as the overuse of ESAs has been linked to thromboembolic risks.
2. *Blood Transfusions: Guidelines and Indications*
   The decision to transfuse red blood cells (RBCs) should be guided by a restrictive transfusion strategy, maintaining a hemoglobin threshold of 7–8 g/dL in hemodynamically stable patients, as supported by current guidelines [3].
   - Over-transfusion should be avoided due to risks such as immunomodulation and increased infection rates.
   - Individualized assessment, incorporating patient-specific factors such as symptomatic anemia and ongoing bleeding, is critical.

7 Coagulation Management

1. *Anticoagulation Protocols*
   Evidence-based protocols stress the need to balance bleeding risks and thrombotic risks in patients who may need anticoagulation after surgery (e.g., those with artificial heart valves or atrial fibrillation).
2. *Restarting anticoagulation*
   Current guidelines suggest reinitiating anticoagulation within 24–72 h post-surgery, depending on bleeding risk [30].
3. *Bridging therapy*:
   In high-risk patients, low molecular weight heparin (LMWH) may be used as a bridge until therapeutic oral anticoagulation levels are achieved.
4. *Managing Bleeding Complications*
   - Correction of coagulopathies using fresh frozen plasma (FFP), platelet transfusions, or specific agents such as prothrombin complex concentrates (PCCs) [37].
   - Antifibrinolytic agents (e.g., tranexamic acid) to reduce excessive fibrinolysis and blood loss, as evidenced by randomized trials [4].

Addressing Thrombocytopenia and Related Concerns:

1. *Platelet Transfusion*: Platelet transfusion is needed when platelet count falls below 50,000/μL in patients suffering from active bleeding or those who had invasive operations [33].
2. *HIT Management*: To manage HIT, discontinue heparin and switch to argatroban or fondaparinux [21, 22].
3. *Refractory Thrombocytopenia*: Investigating and addressing underlying causes, including bone marrow suppression or sepsis, is essential for effective management.

8 Management of Patients with Preexisting Hematologic Disorders Undergoing Cardiac Surgery

8.1 Implications of Anticoagulant Therapies in Postoperative Care

Patients with preexisting hematologic disorders often require anticoagulant therapies, such as warfarin or direct oral anticoagulants (DOACs). Key considerations include:

1. *Perioperative Bridging Therapy*
   - Bridging therapy with low-molecular-weight heparin (LMWH) is typically advised for patients with high thrombotic risk, including those with atrial

fibrillation or mechanical heart valves. This reduces the risk of thromboembolic events after operations and also balances the bleeding risk [45].
- A systematic evaluation by Douketis et al. [5] suggests that the use of LMWH minmizes the risk of serious bleeding in comparison to unfractionated heparin [5].

2. *Resumption of Anticoagulant Therapy*
   - When reinitiating anticoagulants after surgery, it is important to evaluate both thrombotic and bleeding risks. Current guidelines propose that those patients with high thrombotic risk resume anticoagulation within 24–72 h of surgery [29, 30].
   - Monitoring anticoagulation levels is crucial for achieving treatment efficacy without causing hemorrhagic consequences. This is especially important for warfarin and heparin patients.
3. *Reversal of Anticoagulation*
   - Emergency reversal of anticoagulation can be done using vitamin K, prothrombin complex concentrates (PCCs), or andexanet alfa (for factor Xa inhibitors). Studies indicate that these medicines effectively minimize bleeding problems in patients following cardiac surgery [43].

8.2 Management of Antiplatelet Therapy

1. *Perioperative Cessation of Antiplatelet Agents*
   - To lessen the risk of bleeding, patients on dual antiplatelet treatment (DAPT) for coronary artery disease may need to temporarily discontinue medicines like aspirin and clopidogrel. The guidelines suggest that P2Y12 inhibitors like clopidogrel be stopped 5–7 days prior to the surgery, whereas aspirin is frequently continued.
   - Patients at increased risk of having ischemic events may be administered short-acting antiplatelet agents like cangrelor to serve as a bridge therapy.
2. *Postoperative Resumption of Antiplatelet Therapy*
   - Patients at a high risk for thrombosis, antiplatelet medication should be reinstated as soon as possible, generally within 24–48 h. The current evidence shows that early initiation of aspirin following surgery has improved outcomes. Specifically, patients undergoing CABG may benefit most [26, 49].
3. *Management in Patients with Hemophilia or Platelet Disorders*
   - Patients who have hereditary bleeding problems, like von Willebrand disease or hemophilia, need intensive hemostatic support after the operations. Factor replacement treatment or von Willebrand factor concentrates are recommended to maintain adequate coagulation factor levels [46].
   - Antiplatelet therapy should be customized and closely monitored for potential bleeding problems.

9 Case Studies and Challenges in Hematology Management

1. *Thromboelastography (TEG) in Cardiac Surgery*:
   - TEG has proven highly beneficial in guiding blood product administration during cardiac surgery and the early postoperative period [9, 12, 20, 38, 47]. It reduces transfusion rates and improves short-term clinical outcomes by allowing a more precise assessment of coagulation status [20, 38]. Although TEG does not directly influence red blood cell (RBC) transfusion volumes [20], it aids in determining appropriate blood product use, thereby minimizing coagulopathic bleeding and unnecessary transfusions [9, 38]. It also reduces fresh frozen plasma (FFP) usage, minimizing hemodilution [20]. By differentiating surgical bleeding from coagulopathy, TEG helps prevent unnecessary reoperations for postoperative bleeding, even though some studies have not shown a statistically significant reduction in reoperation rates [9, 38].
2. *ROTEM-Guided Blood Product Administration in Pediatric Cardiac Surgery*:
   - A comparative study in neonates and infants undergoing congenital heart surgery with cardiopulmonary bypass (CPB) demonstrated that a ROTEM-based transfusion algorithm leads to more targeted blood product use [28]. This approach reduces total transfusion volumes, improves coagulation, increases hematocrit levels, and decreases postoperative bleeding [28]. ROTEM also lessens the use of additional blood products, including platelets, cryoprecipitate, and recombinant factor VIIa (rFVIIa) [28]. Although FFP use remained unchanged, ROTEM-guided patients showed significantly higher hematocrit levels upon arrival to the Cardiac Intensive Care Unit (CTICU) [28]. With growing clinical experience, ROTEM-guided strategies are expected to minimize unnecessary transfusions, reduce thromboembolic events, and lower costs [28].
   - Further studies in pediatric leukemia patients with leukemia-associated coagulopathy revealed ROTEM's ability to assess and track coagulation abnormalities [25]. Initial ROTEM (EXTEM/INTEM) showed hypocoagulability, while FIBTEM demonstrated hypercoagulability [25]. Over time, coagulation parameters normalized by day 29, with strong correlations between fibrinogen and ROTEM values, emphasizing fibrinogen and platelet count as key determinants of coagulopathy [25].
3. *Systematic Review of TEG/ROTEM in Adult Cardiac Surgery*:
   - A systematic review of 13 randomized controlled trials (RCTs) and six observational studies in adult cardiac surgery patients found that while mortality was lower in the TEG/ROTEM group compared to the control group, the difference was not statistically significant. TEG/ROTEM guidance led to a significant reduction in blood loss and the need for RBC and FFP transfusions. However, no improvement in long-term prognosis was observed. Some stud-

ies showed a reduction in postoperative length of stay (LOS), likely due to fewer reoperations, but no significant impact on 30-day mortality. The use of TEG/ROTEM was associated with a reduction in the volume of blood products used, contributing to cost savings. Notably, TEG testing, which costs around $47 per test, offset these savings through reduced blood product usage.
    - Despite showing consistent benefits in reducing blood loss and transfusion rates, the studies reviewed did not indicate significant improvements in patient outcomes, including mortality, ICU stay, or re-exploration rates. This could be due to a variety of factors such as inconsistent control over surgical variables (e.g., surgery duration, comorbidities), differing transfusion protocols, and the limited sample size in some trials. While TEG/ROTEM may help reduce transfusions and costs, it did not show significant improvements in complications like infection or thrombosis, and more research is needed to evaluate the impact on long-term outcomes and complications [20].
4. *Delayed Recovery of Blood Parameters*
    - Cardiac surgery, particularly with cardiopulmonary bypass (CPB), imposes significant challenges to the hematopoietic system due to factors such as bleeding, blood product transfusion, mechanical trauma to blood cells, hemodilution, shifts in intravascular volume, and the use of anticoagulants and antiplatelet drugs. These factors lead to changes in the three main cellular components of blood. Literature and clinical experience have shown that peripheral blood parameters undergo significant alterations during surgery, with recovery to baseline values generally occurring within 2–6 months after the procedure [15, 17, 34, 35, 44].
    - A prospective cohort study involving 164 patients undergoing on-pump coronary artery bypass grafting (CABG) revealed several key findings. Erythrocytes, hemoglobin, and hematocrit levels declined significantly by day 3 after surgery but gradually returned to normal values within 1 month and baseline levels within 3 months. Leukocytes and neutrophils increased rapidly, peaking on day 2, while lymphocyte counts decreased sharply by day 1. Platelet counts decreased initially but showed a significant increase by day 14, returning to preoperative values within 3 months [16].
    - Postoperative anemia was observed in 100% of the patients, with 32.3% experiencing severe anemia. Anemia is associated with a range of complications, including stroke, myocardial infarction, prolonged hospital stays, and increased mortality. A decrease in hemoglobin (Hb) levels after surgery has been linked to increased cardiovascular events and mortality, as well as postoperative complications like bleeding and platelet dysfunction [16, 23].
    - The study also found that postoperative thrombocytopenia is common, with platelet counts reaching their lowest point around day 2 post-surgery before gradually increasing. Postoperative thrombocytosis, which can

increase the risk of thrombotic events, was observed in some patients and typically resolved within 5 weeks. The mean platelet volume (MPV), which is indicative of platelet size and activation, showed significant changes during and after surgery, with higher MPV levels associated with increased risk of adverse events, including myocardial infarction and vein graft disease.

10 Conclusion

Thanks to new developments such as thromboelastography (TEG) and rotational thromboelastometry (ROTEM), patients undergoing cardiac surgeries nowadays are able to benefit from effective, real-time monitoring of their coagulation-related disorders. This enables the medical providers to tailor blood product management more precisely, support patients at risk for excessive bleeding, and mitigate the risk for thromboembolic events associated with increased blood product utilization. Improved outcomes, decreased cost, and increased patient recovery are direct benefits of using specific target ROTEM and TEG at postoperative period. Therefore, it is advisable to set a standard to include these devices in regular treatment of postoperative patients and further developments in the use of these devices should focus on the improvement of the blood transfusion approach and patient care in cardiac surgery.

It is these studies in particular that underline the changes and interrelations of hematological parameters after heart surgery and the significance of monitoring their changes during the postoperative period. The outcomes indicate that detailed analysis of hematological markers can be useful in assessing the likelihood of complications such as bleeding, thromboembolism, or organ failure.

In the future, it will be necessary to fine-tune TEG/ROTEM-guided protocols to determine the most accurate patient-centered approach for blood product resuscitation. A good next step would be a multicenter randomized control trial that compares this approach with traditional clinician-guided transfusion practices. The study's deisgn may be difficult to undertake because of differences in how surgeries are performed at different centers. Nonetheless, this area of research may prove beneficial in enhancing the effective transfusion practice and clinical outcomes following heart surgery.

References

1. Aftabuddin M, Rajbhandhari N, Rahman Z, Islam N, Khan OS. Cardiopulmonary bypass-induced hematological changes in patients undergoing cardiac surgery. Bangladesh Heart J. 2016;30(2):53–7.
2. Alport C, Mazer CD, Hare GM. Coagulation changes and management during cardiac surgery. Anesth Analg. 2019;128(3):602–16. https://doi.org/10.1213/ANE.0000000000003818.
3. Carson JL, Carless PA, Hebert PC. Outcomes using lower vs higher hemoglobin thresholds for red blood cell transfusion. JAMA. 2016;316(19):2025–35. https://doi.org/10.1001/jama.2016.9185.

4. CRASH-2 Trial Collaborators. The importance of early treatment with tranexamic acid in bleeding trauma patients: an exploratory analysis of the CRASH-2 randomized controlled trial. Lancet. 2017;377(9771):1096–101. https://doi.org/10.1016/S0140-6736(11)60278-X.
5. Douketis JD, Spyropoulos AC, Kaatz S, et al. Perioperative management of anticoagulant and antiplatelet therapy. J Thromb Haemost. 2019;17(8):1331–46.
6. Ezekowitz JA, McAlister FA, Armstrong PW. Iron supplementation and anemia management after cardiac surgery: a systematic review. Circulation. 2020;125(1):97–107.
7. Faraoni D, Van der Linden P. Anticoagulation management during cardiopulmonary bypass: an update. Eur J Anaesthesiol. 2021;38(8):739–50. https://doi.org/10.1097/EJA.0000000000001405.
8. Görlinger K, Pérez-Ferrer A, Dirkmann D, et al. Perioperative coagulation management in cardiac surgery: an update. CME J. 2021;99(6):2563–75. https://doi.org/10.1097/CME-2021-0077.
9. Haensig M, Kempfert J, Kempfert PM, Girdauskas E, Borger MA, Lehmann S. Thrombelastometry guided blood-component therapy after cardiac surgery: a randomized study. BMC Anesthesiol. 2019;19(1):201. https://doi.org/10.1186/s12871-019-0875-7.
10. Liu HM, Tang XS, Yu H, Yu H. The efficacy of intravenous iron for treatment of anemia before cardiac surgery: An updated systematic review and meta-analysis with trial sequential analysis. J Cardiothorac Surg. 2023;18(1):16. Published 2023 Jan 11. https://doi.org/10.1186/s13019-023-02119-2.
11. Karkouti K. Anemia and perioperative red blood cell transfusion: a vicious cycle. Anesthesiology. 2012;
12. Karkouti K, Callum JL, Waters JH. Point-of-care hemostatic testing in cardiac surgery. Can J Anesth. 2020;67(12):1843–55. https://doi.org/10.1007/s12630-020-01745-6.
13. Karkouti K, Callum J, Crowther MA, et al. A protocol to reduce transfusion in cardiac surgery: impact of a practice change. Blood Transfus. 2021;19(3):245–53. https://doi.org/10.2450/2021.0032.
14. Koch CG, et al. Red blood cell transfusion and risk of adverse outcomes after cardiac surgery. Ann Thorac Surg. 2008;
15. Kübler A, Glogowski T, Szabo A. Platelet function during and after cardiopulmonary bypass. Platelets. 2022;33(1):5–16.
16. Lako S, Dedej T, Nurka T, Ostreni V, Demiraj A, Xhaxho R, Prifti E. Hematological changes in patients undergoing coronary artery bypass surgery: a prospective study. Med Arch. 2015;69(3):181–6. https://doi.org/10.5455/medarh.2015.69.181-186. Epub 2015 Jun 10
17. Larmann J, Theilmeier G. Perioperative inflammatory response, hemostasis, and tissue damage: a review. Anesth Analg. 2012;114(4):732–46. https://doi.org/10.1213/ANE.0b013e318243f0da.
18. Lasocki S, et al. Postoperative anemia in cardiac surgery: what are the treatments? Ann Thorac Surg. 2017;
19. Levine GN, Bates ER, Bittl JA, et al. ACC/AHA guideline focused update on duration of dual antiplatelet therapy in patients with coronary artery disease. Circulation. 2016;134(10):e123–55.
20. Li C, Zhao Q, Yang K, Jiang L, Yu J. Thromboelastography or rotational thromboelastometry for bleeding management in adults undergoing cardiac surgery: a systematic review with meta-analysis and trial sequential analysis. J Thorac Dis. 2019;11(4):1170–81. https://doi.org/10.21037/jtd.2019.04.39.
21. Linkins L-A, et al. Heparin-induced thrombocytopenia. Blood. 2012a;
22. Linkins LA, Dans AL, Moores LK, et al. Treatment and prevention of heparin-induced thrombocytopenia: American College of Chest Physicians evidence-based clinical practice guidelines. Chest. 2012b;141(2_suppl):e495S–530S.
23. Lobel G, Javidroozi M, Shander A. Risks of anemia in cardiac surgery patients. Semin Cardiothorac Vasc Anesth. 2015;19:288.
24. Loor G, Koch CG, Sabik JF, Li L, Blackstone EH. Implications and management of anemia in cardiac surgery: current state of knowledge. J Thorac Cardiovasc Surg. 2012;144:538.

25. Malik M, Al-Ghafry M, Haimed A, Su J, Lema M, Shore-Lessersson L, Acharya SS. Exploration of rotational thromboelastometry (ROTEM) to characterize the coagulation profiles of newly diagnosed pediatric leukemia patients. Thromb Res. 2024;233:109–18. https://doi.org/10.1016/j.thromres.2023.11.019. Epub 2023 Nov 20
26. Mehta SR, Yusuf S, Peters RJ, et al. Effects of aspirin discontinuation on cardiovascular events after cardiac surgery: results from the POISE-2 trial. Lancet. 2020;395(10228):1569–78.
27. Muñoz M, Gómez-Ramírez S, Martín-Montañez E, Auerbach M. Perioperative anemia management in cardiac surgery: a narrative review. J Cardiothorac Vasc Anesth. 2021;35(6):1697–712.
28. Naguib AN, Carrillo SA, Corridore M, Bigelow AM, Walczak A, Tram NK, Hersey D, Galantowicz M, Tobias JD. A ROTEM-guided algorithm aimed to reduce blood product utilization during neonatal and infant cardiac surgery. J Extra Corpor Technol. 2023;55(2):60–9. https://doi.org/10.1051/ject/2023017. Epub 2023 Jun 28
29. NCS/AHA. Anticoagulation management guidelines after cardiac surgery. National Stroke Association/American Heart Association; 2022a.
30. NCS/AHA. Guidelines on perioperative anticoagulation management. National Stroke Association/American Heart Association; 2022b.
31. Nelson M, Green JD, Spiess BD, Kasirajan V, Nicolato P, Liu H, Meshkin RS. Measurement of blood loss in cardiac surgery: still too much. Ann Thorac Surg. 2018;105:1176.
32. Nguyen Q, Meng E, Berube J, Bergstrom R, Lam W. Preoperative anemia and transfusion in cardiac surgery: a single-centre retrospective study. J Cardiothorac Surg. 2021;
33. NICE. Blood transfusion guidelines. National Institute for Health and Care Excellence; 2021.
34. Paparella D, et al. Platelet activation during cardiopulmonary bypass. Ann Thorac Surg. 2002;
35. Pereira JV, Williams ML, Walker CA. Hemodilution during cardiac surgery and its impact on coagulation: a review. Ann Thorac Surg. 2019;108(1):337–48. https://doi.org/10.1016/j.athoracsur.2018.12.058.
36. Rahe-Meyer N, Solomon C, Hanke AA. Coagulation management with fibrinogen concentrate or cryoprecipitate. Thromb Res. 2015;135(2):220–5. https://doi.org/10.1016/j.thromres.2014.11.022.
37. Ranucci M, Ballotta A, Kandil HI, et al. Patient blood management in cardiac surgery: evidence and recommendations. J Cardiothorac Vasc Anesth. 2022;36(2):561–74.
38. Redfern RE, Fleming K, March RL, Bobulski N, Kuehne M, Chen JT, Moront M. Thrombelastography-directed transfusion in cardiac surgery: impact on postoperative outcomes. Ann Thorac Surg. 2019;107(5):1313–8. https://doi.org/10.1016/j.athoracsur.2019.01.018. Epub 2019 Feb 12
39. Royster RL, Butterworth JF. Antifibrinolytic agents in cardiac surgery. J Cardiothorac Vasc Anesth. 2018;32(2):947–55. https://doi.org/10.1053/j.jvca.2017.06.017.
40. Sehgal H, Sood S, Sehgal S. Hematology after cardiac surgery: a practical approach. Ann Cardiothorac Surg. 2023;21(5):332–45.
41. Sharma V, Srinivasan A, Kumar A. Coagulation pathways in extracorporeal circulation. J Thorac Dis. 2021;13(4):2481–91.
42. Shore-Lesserson L, et al. Thrombocytopenia in cardiac surgery: pathophysiology and management. J Cardiothorac Vasc Anesth. 2021;
43. Siegal DM, Cuker A, Gonsalves CA, et al. Andexanet alfa for the reversal of factor Xa inhibitor activity. N Engl J Med. 2015;373(25):2413–24.
44. Spiess BD, Spence RK, Fenger-Eriksen C. Inflammation, coagulation, and the endothelial injury triad in cardiopulmonary bypass. Ann Thorac Surg. 2020;110(3):1016–25. https://doi.org/10.1016/j.athoracsur.2020.03.070.
45. Spyropoulos AC, Douketis JD. How I treat anticoagulated patients undergoing surgery. Blood. 2018;132(26):2777–85.
46. Srivastava A, Santagostino E, Dougall A, et al. WFH guidelines for the management of hemophilia. Haemophilia. 2020;26(S6):1–158.
47. Tanaka KA, Bolliger D, Tanaka KA. Coagulation and hemostatic management in cardiac surgery. Transfus Med Rev. 2016;30(2):58–67.

48. Warkentin TE, Greinacher A, Koster A. Heparin-induced thrombocytopenia in cardiac surgery: diagnostics and management. J Am Coll Cardiol. 2018;71(17):2005–20.
49. Willems A, van de Velde M, de Hert S. Postoperative coagulation management in cardiac surgery patients. Eur J Anaesthesiol. 2020;37(10):812–21. https://doi.org/10.1097/EJA.0000000000001268.
50. Zaatari G, et al. Blood transfusion in cardiac surgery: risks and management. Crit Care. 2018.

Postoperative Gastroenterology Care After Cardiac Surgery

Adham Aljariri and Anas N. Shallik

1 Introduction

Gastrointestinal complications following cardiac surgery occur in 0.3% to 2% of cases, ranging from relatively simple issues like paralytic ileus or constipation to life-threatening conditions such as gastrointestinal hemorrhage, with mortality rates ranging from 10% to 60%.

Effective preoperative risk assessment, along with careful intraoperative and postoperative management, is crucial in minimizing the risk of these complications in cardiac surgery patients. Several risk factors contribute to GI tract complications, including hypoperfusion of the splanchnic bed, sympathetic neuronal derangement, inflammatory mediators, opioid use, electrolyte imbalances before and after surgery, and the use of anticoagulation and antiplatelet therapies.

Treatment options vary, ranging from medical management and modification of modifiable risk factors to active interventions such as endoscopic bleeding control and surgical abdominal exploration [1–3].

2 Risk Factors

Several factors can influence the management and prognosis of Gastroenterological complications post-cardiac surgery. Positive end-expiratory pressure (PEEP) is known to reduce venous return, which can complicate hemodynamic stability. Key risk factors include the need for inotropic support and intra-aortic balloon pump

A. Aljariri (✉)
Otolaryngology Department, Ambulatory Care Center, Hamad Medical Corporation, Doha, Qatar

A. N. Shallik
Royal College of Surgeons in Ireland Medical University of Bahrain, Manamah, Bahrain

E. Elmistekawy, N. A. Shallik (eds.), *Perioperative Care of Cardiac Surgery Patients*, https://doi.org/10.1007/978-3-032-09817-7_7

support, which may be required to maintain cardiac output. Arrhythmias also pose a significant risk, potentially exacerbating cardiovascular instability. Preexisting renal dysfunction, indicated by creatinine levels exceeding 125 mmol/L, or established renal failure, adds complexity to fluid and electrolyte management. Similarly, hepatic dysfunction, signaled by elevated bilirubin levels above 14 mmol/L, can impair drug metabolism and increase the risk of complications. Prolonged operation times and protracted ventilation, especially beyond 24 hours, further complicate the clinical picture, often leading to ventilator-associated complications and prolonged recovery times [1, 2, 4].

3 Complications

3.1 Constipation/Ileus

Postoperative ileus (POI) or postoperative dysfunction is a known postoperative complication, it can be linked to perioperative morbidity (enteral feeding delayed, patient discomfort, delayed mobility, and opioid analgesia).

Symptoms can range from abdominal tenderness and bloating to nausea, vomiting, constipation, and obstipation [2, 3].

Enhanced Recovery After Surgery and Perioperative Joint Consensus in 2018 considered a scoring system based on the clinical symptoms.

I-FEED (Intake, Feeling nauseated, Emesis, Physical Exam, and duration of symptoms).

I FEED Score

- Normal, I-FEED score (0–2), tolerating diet with mild nausea in the first 48 hours postoperatively.
- Postoperative GI intolerance, I-FEED score [3–5], nausea, small amount of emesis, abdominal distention, with or without bowel movement, with the first 48 hours postoperatively, most of those patients can tolerate diet and they do not require NG (nasogastric tube).
- Postoperative GI dysfunction, I-FEED score (>6), patients experience severe abdominal pain with distention. No bowel movements and persistent emesis with large volume.

Many treatment options have been proposed for the treatment of POI and POGD including 5HT4R agonists (e.g., Prucalopride), vagus nerve stimulator, prokinetic agents (Ulimovelin), non-drug approaches as coffee and nicotine; however, care must be taken to their potential effect on cardiac dynamics as it may increase heart rate and blood pressure, in addition that chronic smokers may have nicotine receptors desensitization [2, 5].

3.2 Acute Cholecystitis

Acute cholecystitis is a rare complication that occurs in 1% of critically ill patients. The incidence in post-cardiac surgery is reported to be 0.3% ~ 0.7% [6, 7]. Despite relatively low incidence, it is associated with relatively high mortality ~13.7%,

Several factors can be involved in developing acute cholecystitis such as intraoperative ischemia and cholestasis, data has shown that circulatory arrest and intraoperative massive transfusion are predictors of acute cholecystitis, other contributing risk factors Peripheral vascular disease, decreased oxygen delivery, longer times on Cardiopulmonary bypass, surgical reexploration, cardiac arrhythmia, prolonged mechanical ventilation, bacteremia, and nosocomial infections [6, 7].

Diagnosis can be challenging, as the symptoms usually are masked by sedatives, analgesia, and neurologic complications, in addition to delayed onset and nonspecific symptoms. In cardiac surgery, acute cholecystitis occurs late and often asymptomatic, while associated with high mortality, this makes the diagnosis challenging.

It occurs more frequently in aortic dissection surgery group [7].

3.3 Acute Pancreatitis

Occurs at about 0.4% and up to 5.9% after heart valve surgery, it increases postoperative hospital stay and increases hospital mortality.

Risk factors include Hypertension, Chronic kidney disease, History of alcohol abuse, increase cardiopulmonary bypass time, increase cross clamp time, and peri-operative use of epinephrine.

Diagnosis can be based on labs alone, radiologic findings alone, or autopsy findings, but in the majority, it is combination of these criteria. These variations in diagnostic criteria lead to discrepancy of reports of post-cardiac surgery pancreatitis [8, 9].

3.4 Intestinal Ischemia

It occurs in less than 0.1%, but it is severe and associated with high mortality more than 50%, occur often due to non-occlusive mesenteric ischemia (NOMI), it is due to multiple factors such as decrease cardiac output, use of vasopressors on the background of atherosclerosis. It is rarely due to thrombosis or thromboembolism.

Other preoperative identified risk factors include alcohol use and NYHA class 4. Postoperative organ failure marked by elevated creatinine >200 μmol, cerebrovascular incident, use of intra-aortic balloon pump is also linked to postoperative intestinal ischemia.

Incidence decreased after 1996, due to improved perioperative care.

Diagnosis is very challenging as clinical symptoms are masked by prolonged ventilation and sedation, and there is no specific lab test or diagnostic radiologic criteria for bowel ischemia.

Management is mainly supportive, addressing the underlying cause [10, 11].

3.5 GI Hemorrhage

The most common GI complications post-cardiac surgery, compromising 31% of all GI complications, upper GI bleeding is more common than lower. Mortality can reach up to 40% [10].

Duodenal ulcer is the most common cause of bleeding post-cardiac surgery, followed by gastric ulcers, gastric and duodenal erosions, and Mallory-Weiss tears. Factors attributed to GI Hemorrhage are preoperative use of anticoagulation and antiplatelets, intraoperative hypoperfusion that can lead to duodenal ischemia and increase the bleeding risk, increase age, heart failure and chronic kidney disease are among the identified risk factors [12, 13].

H. pylori has a small role of GI bleeding post-cardiac surgery, as studies showed no association [14].

Treatment ranges from medical therapy alone to endoscopic intervention.

4 Treatment and Postoperative Care

4.1 ERAS Cardiac Program

The Enhanced Recovery After Cardiac Surgery (ERAS Cardiac) program comprises evidence-based practices, which was implemented in the United States to improve recovery outcomes in cardiac surgery patients.

It included standardized processes such as preoperative patient education, carbohydrate loading, multimodal opioid-sparing analgesia, goal-directed insulin infusion, and a strict bowel regimen. A comparison of outcomes before and after the program's implementation showed significant improvements (Table 1).

Overall, the program led to faster recovery, cost savings, and higher patient and staff satisfaction.

The key intervention that was implemented in ERAS cardiac program was

- *Preoperative patient education*
- *Carbohydrate loading*
- *Multimodal, opioid-sparing analgesia*
- *Goal-directed perioperative insulin infusion*
- *Thorough bowel regimen*

Table 1 Comparison between outcomes pre- and post-ERAS cardiac program

	Pre- ERAS	Post-ERAS
Postoperative length stays	7 days	6 days
GI complications	6.8%	3.6%
Opioid use	Reduced by 8 mg equivalent	
Reintubation and ICU readmission	Slightly decreased but not statistically significant	
Hyperglycemia	No difference	No difference
Patient satisfaction	86.3%	91.8%

4.2 Carbohydrate Loading

Major cardiac surgery exerts a metabolic stress ad insulin resistance that is worsened by preoperative fasting. It leads to hypoglycemia and reduced insulin sensitivity, catabolic state that increases morbidity, prolongs hospital/ICU stay, and decreases survival. Stress hyperglycemia, even in non-diabetics, stems from the release of glucocorticoids and catecholamines, contributing to oxidative stress and heart damage via glucose toxicity.

Preoperative fasting (for 8 hours preoperatively) aims to reduce aspiration risk during anesthesia but exacerbates surgical stress, leading to postoperative gastrointestinal (GI) issues, delirium, and cognitive dysfunction. Additionally, fasting periods often extend due to logistical challenges, highlighting the importance of minimizing fasting to improve postoperative outcomes and patient satisfaction.

Oral carbohydrate loading typically involves the patient consuming 400–800 mL of oral carbohydrate solution (OCH) the night before surgery, followed by an additional 200–400 mL up to 2 hours before elective surgery. It can be done with other equivalents of fruit-based drinks that are fortified and enriched with nutrients such as glutamine, antioxidants, and vitamins, which do not affect gastric emptying time [15].

Preoperative glucose loading has been shown to reduce insulin resistance and improve glucose metabolism, facilitating a favorable response in the bowel by enhancing its motility and kinetics. However, it should only be used in patients without contraindications, such as gastroesophageal reflux disease (GERD), gastric motility disorders, or gastroparesis [16].

In a meta-analysis by Jonas et al., preoperative oral carbohydrate treatment in patients undergoing elective cardiac surgery was shown to result in a 20% reduction in the use of inotropic drugs, nearly a 50% decrease in ICU stay duration, a 28% reduction in aortic clamping time, and a 35% decrease in postoperative insulin requirements in the cardiac ICU [16].

In two RCTs (Jarvela et al. [17] and Breuer et al. [18]) comparing oral carbohydrate loading (OCH) with overnight fasting or placebo in cardiac surgery patients found no significant differences in glucose levels at anesthesia induction, ICU and hospital stay duration, or the incidence of postoperative nausea and vomiting (PONV). Additionally, there were no significant differences in preoperative hunger, nausea, or mouth dryness between the OCH and placebo or fasting groups. However, patients in the OCH group reported less thirst compared to those who underwent overnight fasting [19].

Other Meta-analysis by Awad et al., showed no statistically significant hospitalization length or postoperative complications among cardiac surgery in patients who received OCH [20].

4.3 Multimodal, Opioid-Sparing Analgesia

Postoperative pain following cardiac surgery (sternotomy) peaks within 48 hours and requires strong effective analgesia to prevent the development of chronic pain.

Table 2 Layers of pain in patient post-cardiac surgery

Superficial	Skin incisions Drainage and dissection/puncture sites (drains, tubes)	
Musculoskeletal	Sternal and costal fractures Sternoclavicular and acromioclavicular joints Zygapophyseal, costovertebral, and cervicothoracic joints	
Visceral	Pericardium Pleura Myocardium (ischemia) Diaphragm	Central through vagus nerve, cervical sympathetic chain, and upper-thoracic sympathetic ganglia.
Neurologic	Peripheral nerve injury (radial, saphenous) Nervous confinement Nervous plexus injury (brachial)	

Although opioids are widely used for postoperative pain, they are associated with risks, side effects and dependency. Since pain may have somatic, visceral, or neuropathic origins, reducing dependency on opioids is essential. Multimodal analgesia, which integrates various medications and regional anesthesia techniques, is recommended to enhance pain management, limit opioid use, and improve surgical outcomes. This approach commonly includes acetaminophen, gabapentin, NMDA antagonists, alpha-2 agonists, intravenous lidocaine, anti-inflammatory drugs, and regional anesthesia [21, 22].

Reducing opioids poses a challenge for both patients and health care providers, as it may confer inadequate pain control postoperatively, it can lead to chronic pain syndrome, increased morbidity, continuous opioid use, reduced functional status and quality of life, delayed recovery time, and increased burden on health care systems [23].

Layers of pain post-cardiac surgery is shown in Table 2.

Opioid-sparing analgesia options following cardiac surgery include paracetamol, gabapentin, NMDA receptor antagonists, $\alpha 2$ agonists, dexamethasone, nonsteroidal anti-inflammatory drugs (NSAIDs), intravenous lidocaine, and regional analgesia. A detailed discussion of the pros, cons, and side effects of each drug is beyond the scope of this chapter.

4.4 Goal-Directed Perioperative Insulin Infusion

Hyperglycemia is a typical metabolic response to trauma, initially triggered by an acute rise in catecholamines, followed by increased levels of ACTH, cortisol, and growth hormone. Pain stimuli can further contribute to hyperglycemia by elevating catecholamines, cortisol, and growth hormone levels.

Table 3 Recommendation of ERAS after cardiac surgery in postoperative phase

Early extubating [22]	Extubating once medically fit, when hemodynamic and pulmonary fit All sedation and pulmonary support should be stopped
Pulmonary function test optimization [26]	Spirometry every 2 hours while awake Head elevation 30° while sleeping Ambulation if tolerated
Multimodal analgesia [22]	Paracetamol 1000 mg Q6h Gabapentin 300 mg BID for 5 days Oxycodone 5–10 mg Q4h (orally or through NG tube) Fentanyl IV for severe breakthrough pain Low dose Gabapentin (100 mg) can be given as maintenance dose in some patients
PONV prophylaxis [27]	Ondansetron 8 mg IV Q4h Promethazine 6.25–12.5 mg given for persistent nausea, avoid for patients more than 70 years old
Bowel mobility [22]	Docusate 100 mg once daily pm Lactulose 20-g solution—If no bowel movement within 48 hours Bisacodyl 10 mg suppository
Glycemic control [28]	Target range 110–150 mg postoperatively
Diet [22, 29]	Ice chips then update as tolerated Chewing gum to enhance bowel mobility
Early mobilization [22]	Once stable and extubated, ambulation 4 times daily out of the bed, 4 times daily as tolerated
Lines and drains [22]	Protocols are established to ensure the early removal of orogastric/nasogastric tubes, central venous lines, invasive hemodynamic monitors, urinary catheters, chest tubes, and epicardial pacing wires

Heparinization contributes to hyperglycemia through the activation of lipoprotein lipase, leading to increased free fatty acids, among other mechanisms. Additionally, hypothermia, rewarming, and cardioplegia also play significant roles in perioperative hyperglycemia.

Target range for blood glucoses are 110–150 mg/d, with treatment algorithms standardized for optimum glycemic control postoperatively [24].

4.5 Thorough Bowel Regimen

Through early mobilization, patients are encouraged to gradually resume activity to promote recovery. Once extubated, they are provided with ice chips, followed by gum chewing and a diet upgrade as tolerated after a swallow assessment to ensure safety. To prevent constipation, Docusate 100 mg is administered orally each night starting on postoperative day (POD) 1, and if no bowel movement occurs by POD 2, a 20-g solution of Lactulose is given orally. Additionally, medications such as Ondansetron and Promethazine are used to manage nausea and vomiting, ensuring patient comfort and facilitating recovery [2, 25]. ERAS recommendation after cardiac surgery are shown in Table 3.

References

1. Ohri SK, Velissaris T. Gastrointestinal dysfunction following cardiac surgery. Perfusion. 2006;21(4):215–23.
2. Mazzotta E, et al. Postoperative ileus and postoperative gastrointestinal tract dysfunction: pathogenic mechanisms and novel treatment strategies beyond colorectal enhanced recovery after surgery protocols. Front Pharmacol. 2020;11:583422.
3. Goettsch WG, et al. In-hospital use of opioids increases rate of coded postoperative paralytic ileus. Pharmacoepidemiol Drug Saf. 2007;16(6):668–74.
4. Schwarzova K, et al. Gastrointestinal complications after cardiac surgery. Trauma Surg Acute Care Open. 2024;9(1):e001324.
5. Arastoo S, et al. Acute and chronic sympathomimetic effects of e-cigarette and tobacco cigarette smoking: role of nicotine and non-nicotine constituents. Am J Physiol-Heart Circ Physiol. 2020;319(2):H262–70.
6. Kamei J, et al. Incidence and risk factors of acute cholecystitis after cardiovascular surgery. Gen Thorac Cardiovasc Surg. 2022;70:1–8.
7. Rady MY, Kodavatiganti R, Ryan T. Perioperative predictors of acute cholecystitis after cardiovascular surgery. Chest. 1998;114(1):76–84.
8. Perez A, et al. Risk factors and outcomes of pancreatitis after open heart surgery. Am J Surg. 2005;190(3):401–5.
9. Chung JW, et al. Clinical implications and risk factors of acute pancreatitis after cardiac valve surgery. Yonsei Med J. 2013;54(1):154–9.
10. Nilsson J, Hansson E, Andersson B. Intestinal ischemia after cardiac surgery: analysis of a large registry. J Cardiothorac Surg. 2013;8:1–7.
11. Pang PYK, et al. Outcome and survival analysis of intestinal ischaemia following cardiac surgery. Interact Cardiovasc Thorac Surg. 2012;15(2):215–8.
12. Mishra V, et al. The correlation between bowel complications and cardiac surgery. Scand J Surg. 2021;110(2):187–92.
13. Krawiec F, et al. Duodenal ulcers are a major cause of gastrointestinal bleeding after cardiac surgery. J Thorac Cardiovasc Surg. 2017;154(1):181–8.
14. Halm U, et al. Helicobacter pylori infection: a risk factor for upper gastrointestinal bleeding after cardiac surgery? Crit Care Med. 2000;28(1):110–3.
15. Tran S, et al. Preoperative carbohydrate loading in patients undergoing coronary artery bypass or spinal surgery. Anesth Analg. 2013;117(2):305–13.
16. Jonas AT, Ljungqvist O. Preoperative oral carbohydrate nutrition: an update. Curr Opin Clin Nutr Metab Care. 2001;4(4):255–9.
17. Järvelä K, Maaranen P, Sisto T. Pre-operative oral carbohydrate treatment before coronary artery bypass surgery. Acta Anaesthesiol Scand. 2008;52:793–7.
18. Breuer J-P, von Dossow V, von Heymann C, Griesbach M, von Schickfus M, Mackh E, Hacker C, Elgeti U, Konertz W, Wernecke KD, et al. Preoperative oral carbohydrate administration to ASA III-IV patients undergoing elective cardiac surgery. Anesth Analg. 2006;103:1099–108.
19. Li L, et al. Preoperative carbohydrate loading for elective surgery: a systematic review and meta-analysis. Surg Today. 2012;42:613–24.
20. Awad S, et al. A meta-analysis of randomised controlled trials on preoperative oral carbohydrate treatment in elective surgery. Clin Nutr. 2013;32(1):34–44.
21. Fernandes RM, et al. Multimodal analgesia strategies for cardiac surgery: a literature review. Heart. 2024;5(3):349–64.
22. Noss C, et al. Enhanced recovery for cardiac surgery. J Cardiothorac Vasc Anesth. 2018;32(6):2760–70.
23. Gan TJ. Poorly controlled postoperative pain: prevalence, consequences, and prevention. J Pain Res. 2017;Volume 10:2287–98.
24. Redant S, et al. Glucose homeostasis during the perioperative period of cardiac surgery: a narrative review. Cardiol Cardiovasc Med. 2021;5(1):36–46.

25. Williams JB, et al. One-year results from the first US-based enhanced recovery after cardiac surgery (ERAS Cardiac) program. J Thorac Cardiovasc Surg. 2019;157(5):1881–8.
26. Franklin E, Anjum F. Incentive spirometer and inspiratory muscle training. In: StatPearls [Internet]. StatPearls Publishing; 2023.
27. Elvir-Lazo OL, et al. Management strategies for the treatment and prevention of postoperative/postdischarge nausea and vomiting: an updated review. F1000Res. 2020;9:F1000-Faculty.
28. Wang Y-y, et al. Postoperative tight glycemic control significantly reduces postoperative infection rates in patients undergoing surgery: a meta-analysis. BMC Endocr Disord. 2018;18:1–12.
29. Noble EJ, et al. Gum chewing reduces postoperative ileus? A systematic review and meta-analysis. Int J Surg. 2009;7(2):100–5.

Everyday Practice in Blood Glucose Management During Perioperative Cardiac Surgery

Mohamed A. Elarref, Walaa M. Hassan, and Noran M. Elarif

1 Introduction

Diabetes mellitus (DM) is a serious medical challenge of the twenty-first century. Persistently elevated glucose concentrations above the physiological range result in the manifestation of diabetes. The peptide hormone insulin released from pancreatic cells maintains normal blood glucose levels by regulating whole body carbohydrate, lipid, and protein metabolism. Insulin performs its function through multiple signal transduction pathways in insulin-responsive tissues, specifically the liver, skeletal muscles, and adipose tissues, which in return form a significant role in the regulation of metabolic homeostasis [1].

Most patients with diabetes experience worsening glycemic control due to the stress of surgery and anesthesia or the use of corticosteroids and nutritional support. On the other hand 40% to 60% of patients without a history of diabetes experience transient hyperglycemia due to the stress of surgery, which resolves in many patients at the time of discharge. Another group of patients with inpatient hyperglycemia are accidentally discovered during hospitalization. Thus, all patients admitted to the hospital should undergo laboratory glucose testing [2].

M. A. Elarref (✉)
Anaesthesia, ICU and Perioperative Medicine Department, HMC, Doha, Qatar

Clinical Anaesthesiology Department, Weill Cornell Medical College in Qatar, Doha, Qatar

Emeritus Professor Anesthesiology, Faculty of Medicine, Tanta, TU, Egypt

W. M. Hassan
Anaesthesia, ICU and Perioperative Medicine Department, HMC, Doha, Qatar

N. M. Elarif
National Heart Institute, Cairo, Egypt

E. Elmistekawy, N. A. Shallik (eds.), *Perioperative Care of Cardiac Surgery Patients*, https://doi.org/10.1007/978-3-032-09817-7_8

In patients with hyperglycemia, measurement of hemoglobin A1c (HbA1c) differentiates stress hyperglycemia from diabetes in those who were previously undiagnosed. Accordingly, The American Diabetes Association and Endocrine Society guidelines indicate that patients with hyperglycemia and an HbA1c of 6.5% or higher can be classified as having diabetes. It is important to emphasize, however, that despite a high specificity (100%), the HbA1c cutoff of greater than 6.5% has a poor sensitivity (57%) and its use is limited in patients with hemoglobinopathies, recent blood transfusion, severe kidney or liver disease, high-dose of salicylates, pregnancy, and iron deficiency anemia. Therefore it was highlighted for the importance to identify and track patients with stress hyperglycemia, because up to 60% of patients may have confirmed diabetes after 1 year of follow-up [3].

Recently, multiple discussions rolled around the incidence of morbidities emerging in patients without diabetes who develop stress hyperglycemia during CABG surgery or during intensive care unit (ICU) stay, in comparison with those with previous history [4].

Unfortunately, stress mediators, namely stress hormones and cytokines, and the central nervous system interfere with insulin secretion and action leading to increased hepatic glucose production with reduction in glucose uptake in peripheral tissues. Accordingly, the adverse outcomes which associate hyperglycemia may be attributed to hyperglycemia-induced inflammatory and oxidative stress as well as its prothrombotic and vascular abnormalities [5].

This chapter aims to provide a better understanding and insight for the future interventions of diabetes mellitus in patients during the perioperative period of cardiac surgeries.

2 Stress Effect on the Blood Glucose Level

Maintenance of normoglycemia is essential for normal body active physiology, and is kept in harmony by a dynamic, minute-to-minute regulation of endogenous glucose production from the liver, kidneys, and glucose utilization by peripheral tissues [6].

The process of glucose production is under the control of gluconeogenesis and glycogenolysis. Insulin forms the main regulatory hormone, by inhibiting the hepatic glucose production and stimulating the glucose uptake by peripheral tissues. During prolonged fasting, a reduction in insulin concentration leads to increased lipolysis (fat breakdown) releasing glycerol and to proteolysis (protein breakdown) releasing lactate and amino acids (alanine) that serve as the most important gluconeogenesis precursors [7].

Under normal physiological conditions, excess glucose is polymerized to glycogen, which is mainly stored in the liver and muscle. Glycogenolysis, mediated primarily by glucagon, breaks down glycogen to the individual glucose units for mobilization during times of metabolic need. These steps are mainly dependent on the harmonic interaction between insulin and counter-regulatory hormones [8].

During stress, the release of counter-regulatory hormones (glucagon, catecholamines, cortisol, and growth hormone) antagonizes the action of insulin, leading to increased gluconeogenesis in the liver together with impairment of insulin action in peripheral tissues resulting in hyperglycemia [9].

Glucagon excess counteracts the action of insulin on glucose metabolism by stimulating glycogenolysis and gluconeogenesis. Furthermore, catecholamines stimulate glucagon secretion and inhibit insulin release by pancreatic ß-cells as well as suppression of glucose uptake in peripheral tissues. High levels of circulating corticosteroids have been shown to increase gluconeogenesis and lipolysis with inhibition of insulin release. Moreover, growth hormone increases hepatic glucose production and causes insulin resistance in humans [10].

Moreover the flaring up of pro-inflammatory cytokines, during the stress response, such as tumor necrosis factor α (TNF-α), interleukin (IL)-6, and IL-1, result in increased insulin resistance by interfering with insulin signaling. Thus, stress adversely affects multiple biological processes, resulting in diminished insulin action, and if the pancreas is unable to compensate by increasing insulin production, the net result is the development of hyperglycemia [11].

The presence of hyperglycemia causes the pancreatic ß-cells to develop desensitization (glucose toxicity) resulting in further blunting of insulin secretion and more increasing serum glucose levels. Recently there is an Increasing evidence indicating that development of hyperglycemia leads to the generation of Reactive Oxygen Species (ROS), which affect different biological signaling pathways [12].

ROS are formed from the reduction of molecular oxygen or by oxidation of water resulting in the production of active radicals, such as superoxide anion, hydrogen peroxide, and hydroxyl radical arising mainly in the mitochondria where NADPH oxidase system becomes the major source of ROS production. As in literature, in moderate amounts, ROS are involved in several physiologic processes that produce desired cellular responses. Whereas exceeding the cellular coping capacity, excess ROS, can lead to cellular damage of lipids, membranes, proteins, and DNA, contributing to ß-cell dysfunction and mitochondrial dysfunction, ending by the development and worsening of hyperglycemia [13].

Pathophysiological effect of insulin on the cardiovascular system.

In the early 1920s, Visscher and Muller were probably the first to attribute a positive inotropic effect to insulin in an isolated heart preparation. Yet, proved documents on the effects of insulin on cardiac function and metabolism remain conflicting. Several aspects of the effect of insulin on myocardial function and metabolism have been studied since then [14].

2.1 Insulin Signaling Pathways Regulating Cardiovascular Systems

Insulin signaling is crucial for regulating cellular metabolism, growth, and survival pathways. The heart , relies on insulin signaling to manage myocardial substrate supply and directly affect cardiac muscle metabolism [15, 16].

The relationship between insulin and the cardiovascular system, focus on insulin's multifaceted influence on cardiac function, from metabolic regulation to the development of physiological cardiac hypertrophy thus insulin signaling modulates glucose and fatty acid metabolism in cardiomyocytes, emphasizing its pivotal role in maintaining cardiac energy homeostasis [17].

The human heart demands a significant amount of energy, relying on a steady flow of nutrients and oxygen to keep intracellular ATP levels stable, which is crucial for the constant cycles of heart muscle contraction and relaxation. With mitochondria occupying one-third of the cell volume in cardiac myocytes—the highest mitochondrial content of any cell type—the heart boasts a robust metabolic system [18].

The heart's metabolic versatility allows it to utilize all classes of energy substrates—including carbohydrates, lipids, amino acids, and ketone bodies—for ATP production in the mitochondria. The primary source of this ATP is the mitochondrial oxidation of long-chain fatty acids (LCFAs), which provide about 60–70% of the heart's energy needs. Additionally, glucose contributes around 20%, and lactate accounts for roughly 10% of the energy production under normal physiological conditions. In a healthy heart, mitochondria are mainly fueled by fatty acyl-coenzyme A (CoA) and pyruvate, the primary metabolites of fatty acids and carbohydrates, respectively. This metabolic flexibility is crucial for meeting the heart's energy demands, especially during increased workloads or stress. The cardiac myocytes' reliance on oxidative phosphorylation within the mitochondria underscores the importance of a constant oxygen supply, which is facilitated by a dense network of coronary arteries and capillaries [19].

Additionally, the heart's ability to rapidly adjust to increased energy demands is supported by the dynamic regulation of key enzymes involved in metabolic pathways, such as AMP-activated protein kinase (AMPK) and peroxisome proliferator-activated receptor alpha (PPARα), which play critical roles in maintaining energy homeostasis. Furthermore, during prolonged fasting, the metabolic environment shifts significantly, leading to increased reliance on ketone bodies as an energy source for the heart [20].

As glucose availability diminishes, the liver enhances the production of ketone bodies, particularly β-hydroxybutyrate and acetoacetate, from the oxidation of fatty acids. These ketone bodies become a crucial fuel for the heart due to their efficiency and abundance. The heart adapts to this metabolic shift by upregulating enzymes involved in ketone body utilization, such as 3-oxoacid CoA-transferase and β-hydroxybutyrate dehydrogenase. This adaptation allows the heart to maintain ATP production and function despite the low availability of glucose. Ketone bodies are more oxygen-efficient compared to fatty acids, yielding more ATP per molecule of oxygen consumed, which is advantageous during periods of limited nutrient intake. Thus, ketone bodies support cardiac energy metabolism effectively during prolonged fasting when fatty acid oxidation predominates and glucose is low [11, 21].

2.2 The Insulin Receptor

The insulin receptor belongs to the superfamily receptor tyrosine kinases (RTKs), and is activated by insulin, as well as insulin-like growth factors (IGF1–2). It is a heterotetrametric protein consisting of two extracellular α subunits and two transmembrane β subunits, which are linked together by disulfide bonds. Most RTKs bind directly to signaling proteins. The insulin receptor, however, binds to phosphorylated residues on partner proteins, namely a family of large docking proteins known as the insulin receptor substrate family (IRS1–6), as well as the adapter protein Shc (Src homology 2 domain containing) [22].

2.3 Insulin Receptor Pathways

When insulin binds to the extracellular α subunits of the insulin receptor, a conformational change is induced, which then results in the autophosphorylation of several tyrosine residues present in the β subunits. These form the binding sites for IRS proteins, which contain phosphotyrosine (PTB) binding domains, or for Shc adapter proteins, containing src-homology 2 (SH2) domains. Binding of the insulin receptor to either IRS or Shc forms a platform that allows for the assembly of a signal transduction particle that gives rise to multiple intracellular signaling pathways [23].

Two principle pathways result from the insulin receptor–IRS interaction, the PI3K/AKT (also known as protein kinase B or PKB) pathway, and the Ras/MAPK (also known as extracellular signal regulated kinase or ERK). The PI3K (phosphoinositol 3-kinase) pathway is linked exclusively through IRS and is responsible for most of insulin's metabolic effects in the cell. The MAPK pathway, on the other hand, stems from IRS, as well as Shc, and is involved in the regulation of gene expression and, in cooperation with the PI3K pathway, also regulates cell growth and differentiation [18].

2.4 Insulin Signaling in Vascular Endothelium Regulating Production of NO

Among the most important cardiovascular actions of insulin is the stimulation of increased production of the potent vasodilator nitric oxide (NO) from vascular endothelium. In endothelial cells, endothelial NO synthase (eNOS) catalyzes the conversion of the substrate L-arginine to the products NO and L-citrulline. Classical vasodilators, including acetylcholine, stimulate an increase in intracellular calcium, which promotes the binding of calcium/calmodulin to eNOS. In the presence of a variety of cofactors, this results in dissociation of eNOS from caveolin-1 with subsequent dimerization and activation of eNOS [24].

The insulin-signaling pathway in vascular endothelium that regulates activation of eNOS employs a phosphorylation-dependent mechanism that is completely distinct, separable, and independent from classical-calcium-dependent mechanisms used by G protein-coupled receptors such as the acetylcholine receptor [25].

Recently, in the literature, a complete biochemical signaling pathway leading from the IR to phosphorylation and activation of eNOS has been elucidated in vascular endothelial cells in primary culture. This pathway requires activation of the IR tyrosine kinase, which then phosphorylates IRS-1 leading to binding and activation of PI3K; and subsequent activation of PDK-1, which then phosphorylates and activates Akt, which directly phosphorylates and activates eNOS, leading to increased production of NO within a matter of minutes [26].

2.5 Other Vasodilators

Prostacyclin (PGI2), a metabolite of arachidonic acid produced by cyclooxygenase-1 in endothelial cells, is another endothelial-derived vasodilator. Insulin acutely stimulates production of PGI2 from vascular endothelium. NO can directly suppress activity of cyclooxygenase-1 and decrease both basal and stimulated release of PGI2. However, inhibition of insulin-stimulated NO production using N (G)-nitro-L-arginine methyl ester does not prevent a PGI2 production in endothelial cells. This suggests that insulin has direct actions to stimulate PGI2 production in an NO-independent fashion. Insulin-signaling pathways regulating PGI2 production are yet to be elucidated [27, 28].

2.6 Insulin Signaling in Vascular Endothelium Regulating Production of ET-1 and Adhesion Molecules

Endothelin-1 (ET-1) is a vasoconstrictor secreted by endothelial cells that opposes vasodilator actions of NO. Recent studies in BAEC and in mesenteric vascular beds have demonstrated that insulin and other hormones acutely stimulate the secretion of ET-1 using MAPK-dependent (but not PI3K-dependent) signaling pathways [29].

Endothelial expression of cellular adhesion molecules including intercellular adhesion molecule-1, vascular cell adhesion molecule (VCAM-1), and E-selectin is critical in modulating cell–cell interactions between circulating inflammatory cells and vascular endothelium. Insulin stimulates increased expression of VCAM-1 and E-selectin on endothelium using MAPK-dependent, but not PI3K-dependent, signaling pathways. Blockade of PI3K-dependent pathways enhances the effects of insulin or vascular endothelial growth factor (VEGF) to increase the expression of these adhesion molecules [30].

2.7 Insulin Signaling in Vascular Smooth Muscle

1. Production of NO in vascular smooth muscle cells (VSMC).

In the vasculature, bioavailable NO originates mostly from the endothelium. Endothelial-derived NO diffuses into VSMC where it activates guanylate cyclase to increase cGMP levels that evoke vasorelaxation. However, expression of eNOS, inducible NOS (iNOS), and neuronal NOS mRNA and protein has been detected in VSMCs in certain contexts. This raises the possibility that NO production in VSMCs may act in an autocrine fashion to regulate vasodilator functions [31, 32].

In VSMC, insulin increases NOS (eNOS and iNOS) activity and NO-dependent GMP production. VSMCs express both IR and IGF-IR. Physiological concentrations of insulin stimulate IR auto-phosphorylation in VSMC and result in a rapid increase in cGMP levels by activating eNOS in human VSMCs. Likewise, stimulation of IR/IGF-IR evokes a rapid release of NO in VSMC (as assessed using an NO-selective electrode). Genistein (tyrosine kinase inhibitor) and wortmannin (PI3K inhibitor) both block effects of insulin to stimulate activation of NO in VSMC, suggesting that the IR tyrosine kinase and subsequent activation of PI3K are both necessary for regulation of eNOS or iNOS by insulin in VSMC [33].

2. VSMC contractility.

Insulin attenuates VSMC contractility by regulating agonist-induced increases in cytosolic calcium through voltage-sensitive calcium channels and altering the activity of myosin light chain phosphatases. This may be mediated by signaling molecules including Rho kinase and PKC. RhoA, a small GTP binding protein, plays a key role in agonist-induced VSMC contraction. Rho activation and membrane localization are regulated by geranyl-geranylation and phosphorylation of Rho. Active Rho Arecruits and stimulates ROK-, which then phosphorylates, and inhibits myosin light chain (MLC) phosphatase leading to an increase in levels of phosphorylated MLC and heightened vascular tone [34, 35].

In VSMCs, insulin acutely inhibits geranyl-geranyl transferase, and decreases membrane levels of RhoA. These inhibitory actions of insulin are NO/cGMP-dependent, and may be mediated by cGMP-dependent proteinkinase1(cGKI). Moreover, insulin-activated cGKI interacts with and activates MLC phosphatase [36].

In VSMC, wortmannin (PI3K inhibitor), and small interfering RNA against Akt abrogates the effects of insulin on the RhoA/ROK/MLC phosphatase pathway, whereas expression of constitutively active Akt upregulates cGKI, ROK-, and MLC phosphatase activities. Thus, the PI3K/Akt insulin-signaling pathway in VSMC is likely to mediate decreased contractility [37, 38].

2.8 Vasoconstrictor Actions of Insulin

In addition to vasodilator actions of insulin discussed above, opposing hemodynamic actions of insulin include activation of the sympathetic nervous system and stimulation of secretion of the vasoconstrictor ET-1 from vascular endothelium [39].

2.9 Effects of Insulin on Blood Pressure

As discussed above, insulin has opposing vasodilator and vasoconstrictor actions such that the net hemodynamic effect of insulin on blood pressure is minimal in healthy humans. Indeed, short-term insulin infusion under iso-glycemic·conditions modestly decreases, or has no effect on arterial blood pressure. By contrast, with iv insulin infusion, intraarterial infusion of insulin does not change, or minimally increases limb blood flow. This is most likely because insulin simultaneously stimulates both NO production and ET-1 secretion. In the presence of ET-1 receptor blockade, intra-arterial insulin infusion causes measurable vasodilation [23, 40].

Acute infusion of insulin also promotes sodium retention by enhancing distal tubular sodium reabsorption in normal, and insulin-resistant individuals. However, prolonged hyperinsulinemia during euglycemic glucose clamp conditions results in compensatory natriuresis due to diminished proximal tubular sodium reabsorption and increases in renal plasma flow and glomerular filtration rate in healthy individuals. Due to the small effects on sodium retention and compensatory natriuresis, it is unlikely that renal actions of insulin play an important role in modulating blood pressure acutely [41].

3 Myocardial Structural and Functional Changes in Diabetes: Evidence from Histology, MRI, and Echocardiography Studies

Structural changes: Pathological evidence characterized by myofibrillar hypertrophy with fibrotic strands extending between muscle fibers to cause diffuse myocardial fibrosis first helped distinguish cardiomyocyte damage in diabetes. The advancement in noninvasive imaging techniques has facilitated further delineation and phenotyping of the diabetic heart. Alterations to left ventricular geometry lead to concentric remodeling, hypertrophy and eventually increased mass. Left ventricular hypertrophy in diabetes includes both concentric and eccentric hypertrophy.

Left ventricular concentric remodeling has been shown to have a higher association with cardiovascular mortality than eccentric remodeling on both echocardiographic and CMR studies. Increased left ventricular mass had initially been shown to be associated with a rise in HbA1c levels in a HF population [41].

Using both echocardiography and MRI has been successful in showing an increase in left ventricular mass associated with diabetes independently of other factors. In summary, there is a general trend that shows an increase in left ventricular mass. However, when corrected for body surface area, which doesn't usually exist, additional decrease in stroke volume is expected in concentric remodeling.

Increased left ventricular mass is a known predictor of cardiovascular mortality and morbidity[. CMR T1 mapping pre- and post-contrast allows calculation of myocardial extracellular volume (ECV) which is a factor for diffuse interstitial fibrosis and correlates with pathology samples obtained in patients with heart failure [25, 42].

However, this is contrary to most existing literature on myocardial extracellular volume (ECV) and T1 mapping to date, which has shown increased ECV and native T1 values in T2D compared to healthy controls. Swoboda et al., also showed increased ECV and native T1 relaxation at baseline in T2D, demonstrating that treatment with renin-angiotensin-aldosterone system inhibition led to an improvement in left ventricular ejection fraction and a decrease in myocardial ECV [43, 44].

Functional changes Diabetic cardiomyopathy has mainly been linked with features of diastolic dysfunction. This is especially apparent in asymptomatic individuals as the earliest sign of HF. Most of the evidence in imaging of patients with T2D have not shown a significant decrease in ejection fraction/systolic dysfunction, with the exception of the Strong Heart Study where a direct correlation of ejection fraction was seen associated with HbA1c levels [45, 46].

Diastolic dysfunction is now regarded as the first functional change occurring in diabetic cardiomyopathy. Strain is a measure of tissue deformation. As the ventricle contracts, muscle shortens longitudinally and circumferentially and thickens radially. The application of strain to measure deformation is constrained by a number of complexities when the parameter is measured by echocardiography [47].

Tissue Doppler imaging (TDI) in echocardiography improved the identification of early diastolic dysfunction, and recent developments in strain imaging on CMR has very much improved the sensitivity and accuracy of identifying subclinical diastolic dysfunction in the T2D population.

Measurement of strain using CMR is now considered the gold standard. Strain rate measures the time course of deformation and this can be derived from speckle tracking echocardiography or measured directly from MRI cine images with dedicated software programs of which several are available. Both longitudinal and circumferential strain have been shown to be impaired in T2D [48].

Table 1a,b identifies the larger and more recent studies that have shown early changes in strain in people with diabetes. Global longitudinal strain (GLS) has been shown to be decreased in the diabetic population compared to healthy volunteers in all the studies described across tissue Doppler, speckle tracking echocardiography, and CMR. Additionally, some studies have shown a decrease in radial strain. Meanwhile one study has shown that peak early diastolic strain rate (PEDSR) and peak systolic strain rate are both decreased in diabetes even when compared to obese/overweight nondiabetic controls.

3.1 Cardiovascular Manifestations of Insulin Resistance

Insulin resistance , leads to significant cardiac metabolic disturbances, autonomic dysfunction, subcellular signaling abnormalities, and activation of the renin–angiotensin–aldosterone system. These factors collectively contribute to the progression of diabetic cardiomyopathy and other cardiovascular diseases [49].

Insulin resistance is linked to hypertrophy, fibrosis, diastolic dysfunction, and systolic heart failure, exacerbating the risk of coronary artery disease and heart failure. Understanding the insulin–heart axis is crucial for developing therapeutic strategies to mitigate the cardiovascular complications associated with insulin resistance and diabetes [50].

In insulin-resistant conditions, impairment of shared insulin-signaling pathways in metabolic and cardiovascular tissues contributes to reciprocal relationships between insulin resistance and endothelial dysfunction. Multiple independent and interdependent mechanisms involving glucotoxicity, lipotoxicity, and inflammation contribute to a vicious synergy between insulin resistance and endothelial dysfunction that helps to explain frequent associations between metabolic and cardiovascular diseases exemplified by the metabolic syndrome [51, 52].

1. Cardiac Metabolic Disturbances

In conditions of insulin resistance, associated with an increase in carbohydrate and fat intake, the reduction in cellular ATP production triggers a state of increased ROS production, leading to intracellular oxidative damage within mitochondria. The oxidative stress at the mitochondrial level induces alterations in the functionality of the sarcoplasmic reticulum, resulting in increased proteasome degradation of incorrectly folded proteins [53].

Alterations in mitochondrial function and the sarcoplasmic reticulum therefore induce changes in the functionality of membrane proteins that manage calcium handling. Impaired calcium handling is associated with reduced intracellular calcium uptake and delayed diastolic relaxation. Along with ROS production and endoplasmic reticulum stress, impaired calcium handling promotes subcellular component dysfunction, ultimately causing apoptosis, necrosis, and autophagy [54].

Under normal conditions, insulin and myocardial insulin signaling stimulate the translocation of GLUT4 and CD36 to the myocyte sarcolemma to supply myocardial energy substrates. However, in a state of insulin resistance, GLUT4 is internalized into cells, resulting in a reduction in energy intake from glucose and increased free fatty acid oxidation, leading to reduced cardiac efficiency [55].

2. Autonomic Dysfunction

Diabetes often leads to neurosensorial damage and neuropathy. Specifically, diabetic Cardiac Autonomic Neuropathy (CAN), even in the absence of cardiac disease, appears linked to both left ventricular systolic and predominantly diastolic dysfunction, although isolating its independent role among the numerous factors involved in diabetic cardiomyopathy is challenging. Initially marked by parasympathetic denervation, early stages of diabetic CAN may promote left ventricular hypertrophy due to excessive sympathetic activation, thereby affecting sympathovagal balance and baroreflexes [56, 57].

Additionally, abnormal signaling of norepinephrine may induce myocardial injury and left ventricular remodeling through the cytotoxic effects of heightened catecholamine levels observed in diabetic rat hearts. These effects are potentially mediated by oxidative stress, inflammation, and apoptosis. Conversely, prolonged diabetic CAN-associated sympathetic denervation may impair β-adrenergic signaling, reducing myocardial contractile strength, relaxation kinetics, and diastolic distensibility [58].

Alterations in myocardial neurotransmitters due to CAN also impair myocardial blood flow and directly worsen left ventricular function. In fact, hyperactivation of the sympathetic nervous system induces vessel wall changes, promoting myocyte hypertrophy and apoptosis, interstitial fibrosis, and reduced contractile function. Additionally, hyperinsulinemia can contribute to hypertension through mechanisms such as sodium retention, which increases blood volume and exacerbates cardiovascular stress [59].

3. Subcellular Signaling Abnormalities

Peroxisome proliferator-activated receptor-α (PPARα) and peroxisome proliferator activated receptor gamma coactivator 1α (PGC-1α) are important signal transduction molecules involved in regulating β-oxidation of fatty acids. This pathway modulates the mitochondrial citric acid cycle and electron transport chain. Moreover, the PGC-1β/PPARα pathway is involved in regulating cardiac metabolism, particularly in conditions of insulin resistance. Specifically, in conditions such as heart failure and diabetic cardiomyopathy, PPARα gene expression is downregulated, and the concentrations of PPARα and PGC-1α are reduced. These alterations contribute to metabolic stress, characterized by a reduction in protective substrates, ultimately leading to a greater predisposition to heart failure and diabetic cardiomyopathy [60].

4. Renin–Angiotensin–Aldosterone System

The renin–angiotensin–aldosterone system (RAAS) significantly influences insulin resistance (IR) and its complications, particularly in hyperglycemic conditions. Despite salt and volume excess, RAAS activation is implicated in diabetic cardiomyopathy, while blocking RAAS has been shown to mitigate cardiac damage [61].

In addition to its AT1 and AT2receptors, angiotensin II (Ang-II) interacts with NOX, leading to increased oxidative stress and inflammation through enhanced production of oxidants and free radicals. Furthermore, heightened signaling through Ang-II type 1 receptors and mineralocorticoid receptors in myocardial cells promotes a proinflammatory immune response characterized by increased leukocyte adhesion, cytokine expression, and macrophage infiltration, contributing to chronic cardiac inflammation. In addition to impairing insulin signaling, activation of mineralocorticoid receptors via RAAS triggers the mTOR-S6K1 pathway, which reduces nitric oxide production in cardiovascular tissues. This reduction impairs cardiac relaxation and, over time, leads to vascular and cardiac stiffness, ultimately causing cardiac fibrosis and diastolic dysfunction [62].

5. Inflammation and Maladaptive Immune Response

In conditions of insulin resistance and diabetic disease, both the innate and adaptive immune systems play a fundamental pathophysiological role in the modulation and progression of inflammatory damage that develops at the endothelial level. Moreover, cardiac insulin signaling also appears to be altered by the pro-inflammatory response. Helper T cells seem to be activated, and concomitant activation of macrophage cells is associated with inflammatory cell proliferation and an increase in inflammatory cytokine secretion, leading to impaired insulin signaling. The activated T cells could modulate increased cytokine secretion, and the resultant milieu of pro-inflammatory cytokines, chemokines, and growth factors is an important risk factor for cardiac fibrosis and impaired diastolic relaxation [63].

As mentioned before, acute hyperglycemia results in nuclear factor kB (NF-κB) activation and production of inflammatory cytokines, such as TNF-α, IL-6, and plasminogen activator inhibitor-1, which in turn causes increased vascular permeability in addition to leukocyte and platelet activation. Furthermore, high glucose concentrations have serious catastrophic effects on endothelial function by suppressing formation of nitric oxide and impairing endothelium-dependent flow-mediated dilation as well as abnormalities in hemostasis, including increased platelet activation, adhesion, and aggregation, with reduction of plasma fibrinolytic activity. Parallel to the effects of hyperglycemia in acute coronary syndrome, high free fatty acid levels that rush up in diabetes and stress can also aggravate ischemia/reperfusion damage by limiting the ability of cardiac muscle to uptake glucose for anaerobic metabolism [4].

Several studies have shown that the hormonal and proinflammatory aberrations associated with stress hyperglycemia return to normal after treatment with insulin and resolution of hyperglycemia. Accordingly, the anti-inflammatory, and anti-hyperglycemic effects of insulin are well established, as insulin acts to suppress counter-regulatory hormone, pro-inflammatory transcription factors, and may even suppress the formation of reactive oxidation species [64].

3.2 Perioperative Diabetes Mellitus and Hyperglycemia

Understanding diabetes mellitus and hyperglycemia, during the perioperative period, is essential for providing appropriate patient care.

Hyperglycemia occurs when blood sugar levels are too high, which can happen in both diagnosed and undiagnosed diabetes. Persistent hyperglycemia can damage various organs and systems in the body, leading to complications such as heart disease, kidney failure, and nerve damage [65].

Undiagnosed diabetes is a significant burden. Many people with diabetes are unaware they have the condition, which delays treatment and increases the risk of complications. Data from the International Diabetes Federation (IDF) shows that nearly one in two persons with diabetes did not know they had the disease in 2021 (44.7%). this represents a substantial portion of the total diabetes population, highlighting the need for better screening and awareness. Efforts to improve diabetes detection and management are crucial to reducing the health burden associated with this condition. Regular screening, especially for high-risk groups, and public health initiatives can help identify undiagnosed cases and provide timely intervention [12, 66].

Perioperative hyperglycemia leads to a higher risk of death, length of stay, and postoperative infections. Hypoglycemia can cause brain damage, which can result in death and severe cognitive impairments [2], 10.5% of Americans have diabetes, according to the 2020 National Diabetes Statistics report. About 21.4% of them go undetected. Surgery is more common in patients with diabetes than in those without the disease (Smiley and Umpierrez 2006) [67].

Diabetes increases the risk of coronary artery disease, which is best treated when many vessels are affected by coronary artery bypass grafting (CABG) [4, 5]. Diabetes that goes undiagnosed is common around the world. A patient who has diabetes (fasting blood glucose ≥126 mg/dl or HbA1C >6.5%) but has not yet received a diagnosis is said to have undiagnosed diabetes [68].

Nearly one in two persons with diabetes were not aware that they had the disease in 2021, according to data from the International Diabetes Federation (IDF) [69]. As anticipated, the burden of diabetes, both diagnosed and undiagnosed, is high among patients undergoing heart surgery. Compared to their confirmed diabetic counterparts, cardiac surgery patients with undiagnosed diabetes appeared to have a greater risk of reintubation, extended mechanical ventilation, and mortality [47].

These results may be linked to these patients' lack of preoperative risk assessment, therapy, and recognition. It is acknowledged that certain patients who exhibit perioperative hyperglycemia but do not have a diabetes diagnosis may actually be experiencing "stress hyperglycemia." According to longitudinal studies, a significant percentage of individuals with initial hyperglycemia have been diagnosed with diabetes within a year [70].

3.3 Negative Impact of Hyperglycemia in the Perioperative Period

Patients in this category face increased perioperative risks, including higher morbidity and mortality rates, as well as a notable reduction in long-term survival and a higher likelihood of recurrent angina. Research indicates that effective glycemic management in diabetic patients can reduce perioperative complications and improve both short-term and long-term outcomes. However, despite the growing awareness of the benefits of glycemic control, there are no established guidelines specifically tailored for cardiac surgery regarding optimal glucose levels during the perioperative period or the best strategies to achieve these targets. Doenst et al. conducted a retrospective analysis of 6280 cardiac surgery patients to examine the clinical effects of hyperglycemia on outcomes. They reported that poor glycemic control during the perioperative phase is linked to increased risks of complications and mortality. Hyperglycemia during cardiopulmonary bypass is an independent risk factor for mortality in patients undergoing cardiac surgery [71].

Elevated glucose levels during surgery have been identified as an independent predictor of mortality in both diabetic and nondiabetic patients. In a retrospective analysis, Fish et al. examined the significance of blood glucose levels during and immediately after surgery in predicting complications among 200 coronary artery bypass graft (CABG) patients. They found that postoperative glucose levels exceeding 250 mg/dL were linked to a tenfold increase in complications [72].

Similarly, McAlister et al. conducted a retrospective study on 291 CABG patients and discovered that average glucose levels on the first postoperative day were strongly associated with adverse outcomes [73], Gandhi et al., in their observational study of 409 cardiac surgery patients, also highlighted the harmful effects of elevated intraoperative glucose levels [74].

Anderson and colleagues investigated the impact of elevated fasting blood glucose levels before surgery in a cohort of 1375 CABG patients. Their findings revealed that patients with elevated fasting glucose levels had a 1-year mortality rate twice that of patients with normal fasting glucose levels and comparable to those with diagnosed or suspected diabetes mellitus [7]. Collectively, these findings underscore the notion that elevated fasting glucose levels before surgery, along with persistently high glucose levels during and immediately after cardiac surgery, are associated with increased perioperative morbidity and mortality in both diabetic and nondiabetic patients [75].

3.4 Anesthesia and Surgical Stress Response

The development of stress hyperglycemia is influenced by a complicated interaction among peripheral insulin resistance, circulating cytokines, and counter-regulatory hormones (growth hormone, glucagon, glucocorticoids, and catecholamines. Increased non-insulin-mediated glucose absorption and insulin resistance are caused by abnormalities in post-receptor insulin signaling. Hyperglycemia, oxidative stress, and glucotoxicity are caused by unchecked gluconeogenesis and glycogenolysis [26]. Insulin resistance also promotes lipolysis, which results in the release of free fatty acids. In addition to glucotoxicity, free fatty acids also cause lipotoxicity and inflammation. Stress-induced hyperglycemia is probably a natural adaptive reaction to improve survival odds [52].

It is anticipated that as the tension subsides, the hyperglycemia would go away on its own. This process is often exacerbated by extrinsic glucocorticoid treatment, which is utilized to reduce inflammation, avoid postoperative nausea and vomiting (PONV), and enhance lung function [61].

It's clear that the extent of surgery and type of anesthesia play significant roles in the severity of hyperglycemia. Intraabdominal and intrathoracic procedures, along with general anesthesia, are particularly associated with more severe and persistent hyperglycemia [76]. The adverse effects of uncontrolled hyperglycemia are well-documented, with studies indicating higher mortality and morbidity in patients with new onset hyperglycemia compared to those with preexisting diabetes. However, attempts to completely normalize blood glucose levels have been shown to be harmful, leading to the current recommendation for moderate glycemic control to minimize the risk of hypoglycemia [77].

Recognizing Diabetes and Hyperglycemia during patient assessment, especially in the perioperative setting, is vital to determine whether hyperglycemia is due to:

1. Known Diabetes: Patients diagnosed with diabetes prior to hospitalization.
2. Stress Hyperglycemia: Elevated blood glucose levels caused by physical stress, often seen in hospitalized patients or surgery.
3. Undiagnosed Diabetes: New cases that have not yet been identified [78].

3.5 Diagnostic Criteria for Diabetes (According to the American Diabetes Association)

A diagnosis of diabetes is made if any of the following criteria is met:

1. Fasting Plasma Glucose: Greater than 126 mg/dL (7.0 mmol/L) after fasting for at least 8 hours.
2. Postprandial Plasma Glucose: Greater than 200 mg/dL (11.1 mmol/L) 2 hours after a 75-g oral glucose load.
3. HbA1C: Greater than 6.5%, indicating poor glucose control over the previous 2–3 months.
4. Random Plasma Glucose: Greater than 200 mg/dL (11.1 mmol/L) in a patient with classic symptoms of hyperglycemic crisis [55].

3.6 Recommendations for Hospitalized Patients

The ADA advises checking HbA1C levels in any hospitalized patient with a blood glucose greater than 140 mg/dL (7.77 mmol/L) if an HbA1C test has not been performed in the last 3 months. This helps in diagnosing diabetes and differentiating it from transient stress-induced hyperglycemia.Importance of Recognition: Accurate recognition and differentiation between diabetes and stress hyperglycemia are crucial for tailoring treatment strategies, managing blood sugar levels effectively, and mitigating the risk of perioperative complications. Proper classification can also ensure that patients receive any needed follow-up care or diabetes management post-surgery [10].

3.7 Management of Oral Antihyperglycemic Therapy Preoperatively

Current medication for glycemic control although the treatment of type 2 diabetes may vary across over the world, a large population of type 2 diabetes adults using oral hypoglycemic agents (OHA) for glycemic management. The major risk of these agents is hypoglycemia which is more commonly seen with agents such as the sulfonylureas and the glinides which both promote or stimulate insulin secretion [78]. Because of the risk of hypoglycemia, it is advisable to stop these agents on the day of surgery and to start again when a regular diet can be resumed [42].

3.8 Insulin Treatment Preoperative Management

Insulin is a component of the treatment plan for all patients with type 1 diabetes and certain patients with type 2 diabetes in order to maintain glycemic control. Patients with type 1 diabetes have an absolute insulin shortage, therefore their insulin prescription covers both the basal requirement and expected dietary and unexpected accidental hyperglycemia. To avoid ketosis, these individuals require more insulin even when fasting [79].

According to Mendez and Umpierrez (2013) Patients should receive 80% of their basal insulin dosage the night before and the morning after surgery. In the perioperative fasting state, long-acting insulin analogues such as glargine and detemir do not peak and are unlikely to cause hypoglycemia; [78] Managing insulin doses in patients undergoing surgery, requires adjustments to reduce the risk of hypoglycemia while maintaining adequate glycemic control.

3.8.1 Long-Acting Insulin Analogues (e.g., Glargine, Detemir)

- Characteristics: Do not peak significantly, hence a lower risk of hypoglycemia.
- Recommendations:
  - Reduce the dose by 25% the night before surgery.
  - Reduce the dose by 50% on the day of surgery, if dosed twice daily.

3.8.2 Intermediate-Acting and Premixed Insulins

- Risk: Higher likelihood of hypoglycemia compared to long-acting analogues.
- Recommendations:
  - Reduce the dose by 25–50% the day before and the day of surgery.

3.8.3 Day of Surgery Blood Glucose Management

- If blood glucose > 200 mg/dL (11.11 mmol/L): Administer 50% of the usual dose.
- If blood glucose < 200 mg/dL: Omit the dose entirely.

These strategies aim to balance the prevention of hyperglycemia during surgical stress with the avoidance of hypoglycemia, which is critical during periods of fasting in the perioperative state [11, 21, 80].

3.9 Insulin Pump Perioperative Management

A continuous basal infusion and preprogrammed bolus dosages of insulin are administered via an insulin pump. Insulin pumps are increasingly being utilized to treat type 2 diabetes after formerly being used only to treat type 1 diabetes. From the initial generation of insulin pumps to the second generation of completely automated insulin closed loop pumps, a great deal of research and development has gone into this field. Closed loop pumps are an innovation in which the insulin pump is connected to a continuous glucose monitor (CGM). This allows the insulin infusion to be adjusted according to the glucose level and a particular algorithm. Few hybrid-closed loop systems are currently in research and very fewer are commercially deployed [80].

It's critical to assess and record the device type, infusion site, pump type, formulation, and dosage schedule for patients who are wearing insulin pumps during their preoperative evaluation. If the procedure is elective, an endocrinology consultation is acquired prior to surgery, and the patient is likely to require hospitalization after the treatment.The requirements for the safe perioperative use of continuous subcutaneous insulin infusions are outlined in their most recent guideline. These requirements include the ability to maintain optimal preoperative glycemic control, keep the pump away from the surgical site, properly position the earthing plate and diathermy away from the pump, and start a continuous infusion if necessary (CPOC 2022). CPOC. Guideline for perioperative care for people with diabetes mellitus undergoing elective and emergency surgery [22].

Throughout the preoperative fasting period, the pump maintains the basal dose of insulin. For brief procedures, the basal infusion could be continued during the intraoperative phase while the insulin pump was kept running. Blood glucose levels should be checked hourly in that case. The insulin pump is turned off and an intravenous insulin infusion is used to maintain a target blood glucose level of 140–180 mg/dl (7.7–10 mmol/L) if the procedure is urgent or is expected to take longer than 3 hours [1, 67].

3.10 Beneficial Effects of Glycemic Control on Clinical Outcomes During Surgery

Maintaining glycemic control (≤180 mg/dL) in patients with diabetes undergoing cardiac surgery:

- Lowers mortality rates
- Reduces morbidity

- Decreases the likelihood of wound infections
- Shortens hospital stays
- Improves long-term survival

A pivotal study by Furnary and colleagues [81] explored the impact of glycemic management on outcomes of 3554 patients undergoing coronary artery bypass grafting (CABG) from 1987 to 2001. The patients were separated into three groups according to the surgery period, glycemic control method, and target glucose levels. Via subcutaneous insulin every 4-hour between 1987 and 1991, glucose was kept below 200 mg/dL. They were treated with continuous intravenous infusion of insulin (from 1991 to 1998) with goals of glucose 150–200 mg/dL. From 1998 to 2001, continuous infusion of insulin maintaining glucose between 100 and 150 mg/dL was adopted as the Portland protocol. This treatment resulted in much lower mean glucose than intermittent subcutaneous insulin. After 1992, the perioperative mortality rate for diabetic CABG patients dropped by 50% (from 4.5% to 1.9%; $p < 0.0001$) with the adoption of continuous insulin protocols, aligning closely with the mortality rate of nondiabetic CABG patients. Additionally, the incidence of deep sternal wound infections significantly declined ($p < 0.001$) [82].

Further evidence supporting the role of insulin therapy for diabetic CABG patient was reported by Lazar and coworkers. In this study involving 141 diabetic patients undergoing CABG surgery, participants were randomly assigned to either a glucose-insulin-potassium regimen to maintain serum glucose levels between 120 and 180 mg/dL, or a sliding scale insulin regimen to keep glucose levels below 250 mg/dL. The glucose-insulin-potassium treatment began at the induction of anesthesia and continued for 12 hours in the ICU. Patients receiving this treatment achieved significantly better glycemic control both immediately before cardiopulmonary bypass (169 mg/dL vs. 209 mg/dL; $p < 0.0001$) and after 12 hours in the ICU (134 mg/dL vs. 266 mg/dL; $p < 0.0001$). Those with tighter glycemic control had higher cardiac indices ($p < 0.0001$), required less inotropic support ($p < 0.05$) and pacing ($p < 0.05$), and experienced fewer infections (0% vs. 13%; $p < 0.01$) and atrial fibrillation (15% vs. 60%; $p = 0.007$). This led to a shorter hospital stay (6.5 days vs. 9.2 days; $p = 0.0003$) [48].

The critical role of stringent glycemic control in patients undergoing CABG surgery was further highlighted in a study by Van den Berghe and colleagues, which included 1548 ventilated patients in a surgical ICU. In this prospective, randomized study, 62% of the patients had undergone cardiac surgery, and only 13% had a history of diabetes. During their ICU stay, patients were assigned to either a conventional therapy group, where insulin was given only if serum glucose exceeded 215 mg/dL to maintain a target of 180 to 200 mg/dL, or an intensive therapy group, which received continuous insulin infusion to keep glucose levels between 80 and 110 mg/dL. Intensive insulin therapy led to a significant reduction in mortality (10% vs 20%; $p = 0.005$), particularly in patients requiring more than 5 days of ICU care with multiorgan failure and sepsis. Cardiac surgical mortality was notably reduced only in patients who required ICU care for more than 3 days. Overall hospital mortality for all cardiac surgical patients, regardless of their ICU stay duration, decreased from 5.1% to 2.1% ($p < 0.05$). Intensive glycemic control did not impact morbidity and mortality in patients with ICU stays of 3 days or less [83].

To further identify which patients might benefit most from strict glycemic control, D'Alessandro and colleagues examined its effect on expected Euro Score outcomes in CABG patients with diabetes. They compared 300 diabetic patients undergoing CABG surgery from January 2003 to June 2004, who received tight glycemic control (150 to 200 mg/dL in the operating room; <140 mg/dL in the ICU), with 300 diabetic CABG patients treated from March 2001 to September 2002, before insulin protocols were implemented, using propensity-based analyses. The group with tight glycemic control had significantly lower observed mortality than expected (1.3% vs. 4.3%; $p < 0.01$), particularly in the higher-risk cohort (EuroScore >4; 2.5% vs. 8.0%; $p < 0.03$). Conversely, there was no difference between observed and expected mortality in the group without tight glycemic control among patients with EuroScore >4 [19].

Two additional studies have highlighted the significance of glycemic control in reducing sternal wound infections. Zerr and colleagues examined the impact of glycemic control on the incidence of sternal wound infections in 1585 diabetic patients undergoing CABG. They found that sternal wound infections increased from 1.3% in patients with average glucose levels of 100 to 150 mg/dL to 6.7% in those with levels of 250 to 300 mg/dL [81].

In another retrospective study involving diabetic CABG patients, Hruska and colleagues discovered that maintaining glucose levels between 120 to 160 mg/dL through continuous insulin infusion significantly reduced the incidence of sternal wound infections compared to intermittent subcutaneous injections [40].

3.11 Glycemic Control in Patients Without Diabetes During Cardiac Surgery

Intraoperative glycemic control using intravenous insulin infusions is not necessary for cardiac surgery patients without diabetes, provided that glucose values remain below 180 mg/dL. Is tight glycemic control necessary for all patients undergoing cardiac surgery? Butterworth and colleagues investigated the effects of tight glycemic control in 381 nondiabetic patients undergoing isolated CABG surgery. In this prospective, randomized study, one group received an insulin infusion when intraoperative glucose levels exceeded 100 mg/dL, while the other group did not receive insulin. The primary outcome measured was the incidence of new neurologic, neuro-ophthalmologic, or neurobehavioral deficits, or neurologic-related deaths. Although intraoperative glucose levels were significantly lower in the insulin group, there was no difference in the incidence of neurologic complications between the two groups. Additionally, there was no difference in operative mortality, need for inotropic support, or length of hospital stay, even though patients without intraoperative insulin had glucose levels exceeding 200 mg/dL. This study concluded that intraoperative glycemic control did not improve short-term or long-term clinical outcomes in nondiabetic patients [14].

Gandhi and colleagues conducted a study on the effects of intensive intraoperative insulin therapy in 400 patients undergoing elective CABG. Participants were randomly assigned to one of two groups: a continuous insulin group aimed at maintaining blood glucose levels between 80 and 100 mg/dL, or a conventional group using intermittent intravenous (IV) insulin boluses to target glucose levels below 200 mg/dL. Diabetes was present in 20% of patients in both groups. The primary outcome, defined as a composite of death, sternal wound infections, prolonged ventilation, cardiac arrhythmias, strokes, and renal failure within 30 days of surgery, showed no significant difference between the two groups. Similarly, no differences were observed in ICU or hospital length of stay. However, there was a trend toward higher rates of death ($p = 0.06$) and strokes ($p = 0.02$) in the intensive insulin group. The study's limitations included the inclusion of patients both with and without diabetes and the administration of intensive insulin therapy to both groups during the immediate postoperative period [35].

3.12 Insulin Infusions Glycemic Control in the Perioperative Period

Continuous insulin infusions to optimize glycemic control in the perioperative period are recommended over intermittent subcutaneous injections or intravenous boluses. For patients with diabetes undergoing cardiac surgery, insulin infusions should be initiated in the operating room and continued for at least 24 hours postoperatively to maintain serum glucose levels below 180 mg/dL. Intravenous insulin therapy is the preferred approach in the perioperative setting due to its ability to allow rapid dose adjustments, which is particularly beneficial during periods of malabsorption, insulin deficiency, or resistance [13].

Various insulin infusion protocols are available, each targeting specific glucose values. Selecting a protocol depends on institutional needs and resources, and its success relies on the comfort and expertise of the healthcare providers implementing it. Protocol effectiveness can be evaluated using metrics such as the time required to reach target glucose levels, specific blood glucose (BG) concentrations, the percentage of values within the target range, or the percentage of time in the desired range assessed through an area under the curve calculation [3, 37, 75].

3.13 Preoperative Management for Patients with Diabetes

Patients taking insulin should hold their nutritional insulin (lispro, aspart, glulisine, or regular) after dinner the evening prior to surgery. Scheduled insulin therapy, using a combination of long-acting and short-acting subcutaneous insulin, or an insulin infusion protocol, should be initiated to achieve glycemic control for in-hospital patients awaiting surgery.

All oral hypoglycemic agents and noninsulin diabetes medications should be held for 24 hours prior to surgery. The hemoglobin A1c (HbA1c) level should be

The hemoglobin A1c (HbA1c) level should be obtained prior to surgery in patients with diabetes or those patients at risk for postoperative hyperglycaemia to characterize the level of preoperative glycemic control.Prior to surgery, it is reasonable to maintain blood glucose concentration 180 mg/d [33]. Efforts should be made to optimize glucose control prior to surgery, because poor preoperative glycemic control has been associated with increased morbidity, including a higher incidence of deep sternal wound infections and prolonged postoperative length of stay infections and prolonged postoperative length of stay [33, 48].

In general, all oral diabetes medications should be withheld within the 24 hours prior to surgery, especially sulfonylureas (e.g., glipizide) and glinides (e.g., nateglinideor repaglinide). These drugs can induce hypoglycemia in the absence of food. Patients who are taking insulin and who are admitted on the day of surgery should be instructed to continue their basal insulin dose (e.g., glargine, detemir, or NPH) and hold their nutritional insulin (e.g., lispro, aspart, glulisine, or regular) unless instructed otherwise by their primary physician. The NPH insulin may be reduced by one half or one third prior to surgery to avoid hypoglycemia. To achieve rapid control in a hospitalized patient with hyperglycemia (glucose persistently 180 mg/dL for 12 hours before surgery), insulin therapy either with intravenous variable-rate continuous infusion or subcutaneous basal plus rapid-acting insulin should be used depending on the availability of either therapy [6, 9].

For patients who are hyperglycemic in the preoperative area on the day of surgery, IV insulin therapy is an effective method for rapid control. Patients with a known history of diabetes (type 1 or type 2) can be started on IV therapy immediately in the preoperative area. It's important to review all preoperative medications to assess the potential for insulin resistance, including steroids, protease inhibitors, and antipsychotic drugs. Additionally, patients with renal insufficiency should be identified, as impaired insulin clearance increases the risk of hypoglycemia. Hemoglobin A1c (HbA1c), a glycosylated hemoglobin, accurately indicates glycemic control over a 2–3 month period. The American Diabetes Association states that adequate glycemic control is associated with an HbA1c of less than 7%. Obtaining an HbA1c prior to surgery in diabetic patients or those at risk for postoperative hyperglycemia helps optimize glycemic control in patients with elevated HbA1c levels and identifies those who may need more aggressive glycemic management upon hospital discharge [6].

3.14 Intraoperative Control Recommendations

Glucose levels above 180 mg/dL in patients without diabetes during cardiopulmonary bypass can initially be treated with a single or intermittent dose of IV insulin, provided levels remain below 180 mg/dL. For patients with persistently elevated serum glucose (above 180 mg/dL) after cardiopulmonary bypass, a continuous insulin drip should be started, and an endocrinology consult should be obtained. If an intravenous insulin infusion is started in the preoperative period, it should continue throughout the intraoperative and early postoperative periods according to institutional protocols to maintain serum glucose below 180 mg/dL [67].

Patients on IV insulin infusions should have their blood glucose monitored every 30 to 60 minutes, with more frequent monitoring (every 15 minutes) during periods of rapidly fluctuating sensitivity, such as during cardioplegia administration and systemic cooling and rewarming. Patients with IV insulin infusions started in the preoperative period should continue them in the operating room to maintain serum glucose below 180 mg/dL. Patients without a history of diabetes may experience transient blood glucose elevations above 180 mg/dL during cardiopulmonary bypass. These patients may have insulin resistance and should be treated with a single or intermittent dose of IV insulin to maintain glucose below 180 mg/dL. Caution is advised when initiating a continuous IV insulin drip in these patients, as insulin requirements may decrease rapidly in the immediate postoperative period, potentially causing serious hypoglycemia [80].

Patients without a prior diagnosis of diabetes but with persistently high glucose levels (≥180 mg/dL) during surgery should receive continuous intravenous (IV) insulin therapy. Since a significant proportion of these patients may later be diagnosed with diabetes, consulting an endocrinologist in the postoperative period is advisable [16].

3.15 Glycemic Control in the ICU

Patients, irrespective of diabetes status, who exhibit persistently elevated glucose levels (≥180 mg/dL) should receive IV insulin infusions to maintain glucose levels below 180 mg/dL throughout their ICU stay [55, 78]. Any patient requiring extended ICU care (≥3 days) due to mechanical ventilation, inotropic or mechanical support, renal replacement therapies, or anti-arrhythmic treatments should also receive continuous IV insulin infusions to target glucose levels below 150 mg/dL. Before discontinuing IV insulin therapy, patients should transition to subcutaneous insulin following institutional protocols [80]. Hourly glucose monitoring should be performed until levels stabilize to reduce fluctuations and minimize hypoglycemia risks, which are rare and associated with minimal adverse effects. Upon ICU discharge, transitioning patients to subcutaneous insulin regimens is critical, with dosing based on insulin usage over the previous 24 hours and nutritional intake [84].

3.16 Glycemic Control on Floors

Postprandial glucose should remain below 180 mg/d, Fasting and pre-meal glucose targets should be below 110 mg/dL after transfer to the floor. Oral diabetes medications can be resumed for patients meeting glucose targets if no contraindications exist, and insulin doses adjusted accordingly [83].

For noncritically ill patients, the American Association of Clinical Endocrinologists recommends a pre-meal glucose target of ≤110 mg/dL and a postprandial or random glucose level ≤180 mg/dL. This control is best achieved using scheduled basal and bolus insulin therapies, such as glargine or detemir (basal) and lispro, aspart, or glulisine (bolus). Patients with type 2 diabetes who were on oral medications preoperatively can restart these medications upon achieving glycemic targets and resuming regular diets. However, metformin should not be reintroduced until renal function stabilizes, and thiazolidinediones (e.g., pioglitazone, rosiglitazone) should only be restarted in patients without heart failure or liver dysfunction [85].

3.17 Preparation for Hospital Discharge

Before discharge, patients with diabetes or those newly initiated on a glycemic control regimen should receive in-hospital education. This education must cover glucose monitoring, medication usage (including insulin injections when needed), nutrition, and lifestyle adjustments.At discharge, updates to the glycemic management plan should be communicated to the patient's primary care provider, and follow-up appointments with an endocrinologist should be scheduled when applicable. Patients experiencing hyperglycemia after cardiac surgery should be evaluated by an inpatient diabetes care team to establish an appropriate post-discharge glycemic management strategy [86].

If hyperglycemia is first identified perioperatively, or if insulin therapy or a new insulin protocol is initiated, specialized education should be provided before discharge. This training, ideally starting at least 2 days before discharge, can be delivered by certified diabetes educators and supported by nurses or registered dietitians skilled in diabetes care. It should include instruction on glucose monitoring, medication administration, diet, physical activity, and lifestyle changes. Arrangements for follow-up care with primary care physicians must be made before discharge, and any modifications to the diabetes management plan should be communicated to the referring providers [44, 81].

4 Conclusion

Hyperglycemia and hypoglycemia significantly affect mortality and morbidity. Proper preoperative evaluation and optimization of diabetic patients are crucial and can enhance perioperative outcomes. Currently, there is no evidence supporting perioperative intensive insulin therapy and strict glucose control in cardiac or noncardiac surgical patients. A moderate glycemic target of maintaining blood glucose between 140 and 180 mg/dl (7.7–10 mmol/L) with conventional insulin therapy leads to fewer hypoglycemic episodes and improved survival.

References

1. Abdelmalak B, Ibrahim M, Yared JP, Modic MB, Nasr C. Perioperative glycemic management in insulin pump patients undergoing noncardiac surgery. Curr Pharm Des. 2012;18(38):6204–14.
2. Abdelmalak BB, Lansang MC. Revisiting tight glycemic control in perioperative and critically ill patients: when one size may not fit all. J Clin Anesth. 2013;25(6):499–507.
3. American Association of Clinical Endocrinologists medical guidelines for clinical practice for the management of diabetes mellitus. Endocr Pract. 2007;13:1–68.
4. Naito R, Miyauchi K. Coronary artery disease and type 2 diabetes mellitus. Int Heart J. 2017;58(4):475–80.
5. American Diabetes Association. 2. Classification and diagnosis of diabetes: standards of medical care in diabetes-2020. Diabetes Care. 2020;43(Suppl 1):S14–31. https://doi.org/10.2337/dc20-S002.
6. American Diabetes Association. 6. Glycemic targets: standards of medical care in diabetes-2020. Diabetes Care. 2020;43(Suppl 1):S66–76.
7. Anderson RE, Brismar K, Barr G, Ivert T. Effects of cardiopulmonary bypass on glucose homeostasis after coronary artery bypass surgery. Eur J Cardiothorac Surg. 2005;28:425–30.
8. Malik A, et al. A study of the anti-diabetic agents of camel milk. Int J Mol Med. 2012;30(3):585–92. https://doi.org/10.3892/ijmm.2012.1051.
9. Association AD. 9. Pharmacologic approaches to glycemic treatment: standards of medical care in diabetes—2021. Diabetes Care. 2021;44(Supplement 1):S111–24.
10. Association AD. 15. Diabetes care in the hospital: standards of medical care in diabetes—2021. Diabetes Care. 2021;44(Supplement 1):S211–20.
11. Barker P, Creasey PE, Dhatariya K, et al. Peri-operative management of the surgical patient with diabetes 2015: Association of Anaesthetists of Great Britain and Ireland. Anaesthesia. 2015;70(12):1427–40.
12. Bodiga VL, Eda SR, Bodiga S. Advanced glycation end products: role in pathology of diabetic cardiomyopathy. Heart Fail Rev. 2014;19:49–63.
13. Braithwaite SS, Godara H, Song HJ, Rock P. No patient left behind: evaluation and design of intravenous insulin infusion algorithms. Endocr Pract. 2006;12:72–8.
14. Butterworth J, Wagenknecht LE, Legault C, et al. Attempted control of hyperglycemia during cardiopulmonary bypass fails to improve neurologic or neurobehavioral outcomes in patients without diabetes mellitus undergoing coronary artery bypass grafting. J Thorac Cardiovasc Surg. 2005;130:1319–23.
15. Christensen RH, Hansen CS, von Scholten BJ, Jensen MT, Pedersen BK, Schnohr P, Vilsbøll T, Rossing P, Jørgensen PG. Epicardial and pericardial adipose tissues are associated with reduced diastolic and systolic function in type 2 diabetes. Diabetes Obes Metab. 2019;21(8):2006–11.
16. CPOC. Guideline for perioperative care for people with diabetes mellitus undergoing elective and emergency surgery. 2022.
17. Critchell CD, Savarese V, Callahan A, Aboud C, Jabbour S, Marik P. Accuracy of bedside capillary blood glucose measurements in critically ill patients. Intensive Care Med. 2007;33(12):2079–84.
18. D'Alessandris C, Lauro R, Presta I, Sesti G. C-reactive protein induces phosphorylation of insulin receptor substrate-1 on Ser307 and Ser 612 in L6 myocytes, thereby impairing the insulin signalling pathway that promotes glucose transport. Diabetologia. 2007;50(4):840–9. https://doi.org/10.1007/s00125-006-0522-y. Epub 2007 Feb 6. PMID: 17279354.
19. D'Alessandro C, Leprince P, Golmard JL, et al. Strict glycemic control reduces EuroSCORE expected mortality in diabetic patients undergoing myocardial revascularization. J Thorac Cardiovasc Surg. 2007;134:29–37.
20. De Ferranti SD, de Boer IH, Fonseca V, Fox CS, Golden SH, Lavie CJ, et al. Type 1 diabetes mellitus and cardiovascular disease: a scientific statement from the American Heart Association and American Diabetes Association. Circulation. 2014;130(13):1110e1130.

21. Demma LJ, Carlson KT, Duggan EW, Morrow JG 3rd, Umpierrez G. Effect of basal insulin dosage on blood glucose concentration in ambulatory surgery patients with type 2 diabetes. J Clin Anesth. 2017;36:184–8.
22. Diabetes-Guideline-Updated2022.pdf (Accessed 30 Dec 2022 2022). https://www.cpoc.org.uk/sites/cpoc/files/documents/2022-12/CPOCf (Accessed 30 Dec 2022).
23. Doenst T, Wijeysundera D, Karkouti K, Zechner C, Maganti M, Rao V, Borger MA. Hyperglycemia during cardiopulmonary bypass is an independent risk factor for mortality in patients undergoing cardiac surgery. J Thorac Cardiovasc Surg. 2005;130(4):1144.e1–8.
24. Ducheix S, Magre J, Cariou B, Prieur X. Chronic O-GlcNAcylation and diabetic cardiomyopathy: the bitterness of glucose. Front Endocrinol. 2018;9:642.
25. Duggan EW, Carlson K, Umpierrez GE. Perioperative hyperglycemia management: an update. Anesthesiology. 2017;126(3):547–60.
26. Dungan KM, Braithwaite SS, Preiser JC. Stress hyperglycaemia. Lancet. 2009;373(9677):1798–807. https://doi.org/10.1016/S0140-6736(09)60553-5.
27. Eelen G, de Zeeuw P, Treps L, Harjes U, Wong BW, Carmeliet P. Endothelial cell metabolism. Physiol Rev. 2018;98(1):3–58.
28. Levelt E, Mahmod M, Piechnik SK, Ariga R. Relationship between left ventricular structural and metabolic remodeling in type 2 diabetes- Diabetes. Am Diabetes Assoc. 2016.
29. Finfer S, Chittock DR, Su SY, et al. Intensive versus conventional glucose control in critically ill patients. N Engl J Med. 2009;360(13):1283–97.
30. Fish LH, Weaver TW, Moore AL, Steel LG. Value of postoperative blood glucose in predicting complications and length of stay after coronary artery bypass grafting. Am J Cardiol. 2003;92:74–6.
31. Frisch A, Chandra P, Smiley D, et al. Prevalence and clinical outcome of hyperglycemia in the perioperative period in noncardiac surgery. Diabetes Care. 2010;33(8):1783–8.
32. Fritsche A, Stumvoll M, Goebbel S, Reinauer KM, Schmulling RM, Haring HU. Long term effect of a structured inpatient diabetes teaching and treatment program in type 2 diabetic patients: influence of mode of follow-up. Diabetes Res Clin Pract. 1999;46:135–41.
33. Furnary AP, Wu Y, Bookin SO. Effect of hyperglycemia and continuous intravenous insulin infusions on outcomes of cardiac surgical procedures: the Portland Diabetic Project. Endocr Pract. 2004;10(2):21–33.
34. Gandhi GY, Nuttall GA, Abel MD, et al. Intraoperative hyperglycemia and perioperative outcomes in cardiac surgery patients. Mayo Clin Proc. 2005;80:862–6.
35. Gandhi GY, Nuttall GA, Abel MD, et al. Intensive intraoperative insulin therapy versus conventional glucose management during cardiac surgery: a randomized trial. Ann Intern Med. 2007;146(4):233–43.
36. Gimbrone MA Jr, Garcia-Cardena G. Endothelial cell dysfunction and the pathobiology of atherosclerosis. Circ Res. 2016;118(4):620e–636.
37. Goldberg PA, Bozzo JE, Thomas PG, et al. "Glucometrics"—assessing the quality of inpatient glucose management. Diabetes Technol Ther. 2006;8:560–9.
38. Gray S, Kim JK. New insights into insulin resistance in the diabetic heart. Trends Endocrinol Metab. 2011;22:394–403.
39. Hasan SS, Jabs M, Taylor J, Wiedmann L, Leibing T, Nordstrom V, et al. Endothelial notch signaling controls insulin transport in muscle. EMBO Mol Med. 2020;12(4):e09271.
40. Hruska LA, Smith JM, Hendy MP, Fritz VL, McAdams S. Continuous insulin infusion reduces infectious complications in diabetics following coronary surgery. J Card Surg. 2005;20:403–7.
41. Fu J, Yu MG, Li Q, et al. Insulin actions on the vascular tissues: physiological effects and pathophysiological contributions to vascular complications of diabetes. Mol Metab. 2021;52(6):101236. https://doi.org/10.1016/j.molmet.2021.101236.
42. Joshi GP, Chung F, Vann MA, et al. Society for ambulatory anesthesia consensus statement on perioperative blood glucose management in diabetic patients undergoing ambulatory surgery. Anesth Analg. 2010;111(6):1378–87.
43. King GL, Park K, Li Q. Selective insulin resistance and the development of cardiovascular diseases in diabetes: the 2015 Edwin Bierman award lecture. Diabetes. 2016;65(6):1462.

44. Ko SH, Song KH, Kim SR, et al. Long-term effects of a structured intensive diabetes education program (SIDEP) in patients with type 2 diabetes mellitus—a 4-year follow-up study. Diabet Med. 2007;24:55–62.
45. Lacolley P, Regnault V, Segers P, Laurent S. Vascular smooth muscle cells and arterial stiffening: relevance in development, aging, and disease. Physiol Rev. 2017;97(4):1555–617.
46. Lang RM, Badano LP, Mor-Avi V, Afilalo J, Armstrong A, Ernande L, Flachskampf FA, Foster E, Goldstein SA, Kuznetsova T, et al. Recommendations for cardiac chamber quantification by echocardiography in adults: an update from the American Society of Echocardiography and the European Association of Cardiovascular Imaging. Eur Heart J Cardiovasc Imaging. 2015;16:233–70.
47. Lauruschkat AH, Arnrich B, Albert AA, et al. Prevalence and risks of undiagnosed diabetes mellitus in patients undergoing coronary artery bypass grafting. Circulation. 2005;112(16):2397–402.
48. Lazar HL, Chipkin SR, Fitzgerald CA, Bao Y, Cabral H, Apstein CS. Tight glycemic control in diabetic coronary artery bypass graft patients improves perioperative outcomes and decreases recurrent ischemic events. Circulation. 2004;109:1497–502.
49. Levy N, Dhatariya K. Pre-operative optimisation of the surgical patient with diagnosed and undiagnosed diabetes: a practical review. Anaesthesia. 2019;74(Suppl 1):58–66.
50. Li Q, Fu J, Xia Y, Qi W, Ishikado A, Park K, et al. Homozygous receptors for insulin and not IGF-1 accelerate intimal hyperplasia in insulin resistance and diabetes. Nat Commun. 2019;10(1):4427.
51. Lipshutz Angela KM, Gropper Michael A, Warner David S, Warner MA. Perioperative glycemic controlan evidence-based review. Anesthesiology. 2009;110(2):408–21.
52. Marik PE, Bellomo R. Stress hyperglycemia: an essential survival response! Crit Care. 2013;17(2):305.
53. Mather KJ, Steinberg HO, Baron AD. Insulin resistance in the vasculature. J Clin Invest. 2013;123(3):1003–4.
54. Matshela M. Second in a series on diabetes and the heart: diabetic cardiomyopathy-mechanisms and mode of diagnosis. E-J Cardiol Pract. 2016:14.
55. Mazurek JA, Hailpern SM, Goring T, Nordin C. Prevalence of hemoglobin A1c greater than 6.5% and 7.0% among hospitalized patients without known diagnosis of diabetes at an urban inner city hospital. J Clin Endocrinol Metab. 2010;95(3):1344–8.
56. McAlister FA, Man J, Bistritz L, Amad H, Tandon P. Diabetes and coronary artery bypass surgery: an examination of perioperative glycemic control and outcomes. Diabetes Care. 2003;26:1518–24.
57. Mellor KM, Bell JR, Young MJ, Ritchie RH, Delbridge LM. Myocardial autophagy activation and suppressed survival signaling is associated with insulin resistance in fructose-fed mice. J Mol Cell Cardiol. 2011;50:1035–43. https://doi.org/10.1016/j.yjmcc.2011.03.002.
58. Mendez CE, Umpierrez G. Management of the hospitalized patient with type 1 diabetes mellitus. Hosp Pract (1995). 2013;41(3):89–100.
59. Højlund K. Metabolism and insulin signaling in common metabolic disorders and inherited insulin resistance. Dan Med J. 2014;61(7):B4890. PMID: 25123125 Review.
60. Zamora M, Villena JA. Contribution of impaired insulin signaling to the pathogenesis of diabetic cardiomyopathy. Int J Mol Sci. 2019;20(11):2833. https://doi.org/10.3390/ijms20112833.
61. Morariu AM, Loef BG, Aarts LP, et al. Dexamethasone: benefit and prejudice for patients undergoing on-pump coronary artery bypass grafting: a study on myocardial, pulmonary, renal, intestinal, and hepatic injury. Chest. 2005;128(4):2677–87.
62. Murphy SP, Kakkar R, McCarthy CP, Januzzi JL. Inflammation in heart failure: JACC state-of-the-art review. J Am Coll Cardiol. 2020;75(11):1324–40.
63. Nagueh SF, Smiseth OA, Appleton CP, Byrd BF III, Dokainish H, Edvardsen T, Flachskampf FA, Gillebert TC, Klein AL, Lancellotti P, et al. Recommendations for the evaluation of left ventricular diastolic function by echocardiography: an update from the American Society of Echocardiography and the European Association of Cardiovascular Imaging. Eur Heart J Cardiovasc Imaging. 2016;17:1321–60.

64. National Diabetes Inpatient Audit- Harms 2022 England. 2021.
65. Lee A, Hakuno F, Northcott P, Pessin JE, Rozakis Adcock M. Nexilin, a cardiomyopathy-associated F-actin binding protein, binds and regulates IRS1 signaling in skeletal muscle cells. PLoS One. 2013;8(1):e55634. https://doi.org/10.1371/journal.pone.0055634. Epub 2013 Jan 30.PMID: 23383252.
66. Ogurtsova K, Guariguata L, Barengo NC, et al. IDF diabetes atlas: global estimates of undiagnosed diabetes in adults for 2021. Diabetes Res Clin Pract. 2022;183:109118.
67. Partridge H, Perkins B, Mathieu S, Nicholls A, Adeniji K. Clinical recommendations in the management of the patient with type 1 diabetes on insulin pump therapy in the perioperative period: a primer for the anaesthetist. Br J Anaesth. 2016;116(1):18–26.
68. De Meyts P, Feingold KR, Anawalt B, Blackman MR, Boyce A, Chrousos G, Corpas E, de Herder WW, Dhatariya K, Dungan K, Hofland J, Kalra S, Kaltsas G, Kapoor N, Koch C, Kopp P, et al. The insulin receptor and its signal transduction network. Endotext [internet]. South Dartmouth (MA): DText.com, Inc; 2016.
69. Swoboda PP, McDiarmid AK, Erhayiem B. Diabetes mellitus, microalbuminuria, and subclinical cardiac disease: identification and monitoring of individuals at risk of heart failure. J Am Heart Assoc. 2017;6:e005539.
70. Ramirez-Correa GA, Ma J, Slawson C, Zeidan Q, Lugo-Fagundo NS, Xu M, Shen X, Gao WD, Caceres V, Chakir K, et al. Removal of abnormal myofilament O-GlcNAcylation restores Ca^{2+} sensitivity in diabetic cardiac muscle. Diabetes. 2015;64:3573–87.
71. Rask-Madsen C, Kahn CR. Tissue-specific insulin signaling, metabolic syndrome, and cardiovascular disease. Arterioscler Thromb Vasc Biol. 2012;32(9):2052e205974.
72. Rawshani A, Rawshani A, Franzen S, Eliasson B, Svensson AM, Miftaraj M, et al. Mortality and cardiovascular disease in type 1 and type 2 diabetes. N Engl J Med. 2017;376(15):1407–18.
73. Sreedharan R, Khanna S, Shaw A. Perioperative glycemic management in adults presenting for elective cardiac and non-cardiac surgery. Perioperative Med. 2023;12:13.
74. Sathya B, Davis R, Taveira T, Whitlatch H, Wu WC. Intensity of peri-operative glycemic control and postoperative outcomes in patients with diabetes: a meta-analysis. Diabetes Res Clin Pract. 2013;102(1):8–15.
75. Schmeltz LR, DeSantis AJ, Schmidt K, et al. Conversion of intravenous insulin infusions to subcutaneously administered insulin glargine in patients with hyperglycemia. Endocr Pract. 2006;12:641–50.
76. Singh LG, Satyarengga M, Marcano I, et al. Reducing inpatient hypoglycemia in the general wards using real-time continuous glucose monitoring: the glucose telemetry system, a randomized clinical trial. Diabetes Care. 2020;43(11):2736–43.
77. Smiley DD, Umpierrez GE. Perioperative glucose control in the diabetic or nondiabetic patient. South Med J. 2006;99(6):580–9. (quiz 90–1).
78. Sreedharan R, Abdelmalak B. Diabetes mellitus: preoperative concerns and evaluation. Anesthesiol Clin. 2018;36(4):581–97.
79. Sousa GR, Pober D, Galderisi A, Lv H, Yu L, Pereira AC, et al. Glycemic control, cardiac autoimmunity, and long-term risk of cardiovascular disease in type 1 diabetes mellitus. Circulation. 2019;139(6):730e–743.
80. Templer S. Closed-loop insulin delivery systems: past, present, and future directions. Front Endocrinol (Lausanne). 2022;13:919942.
81. Zerr KJ, Furnary AP, Grunkemeier GL, Bookin S, Kanhere V, Starr A. Glucose control lowers the risk of wound infection in diabetics after open heart operations. Ann Thorac Surg. 1997;63:356–61.
82. Furnary AP, Cheek DB, Holmes SC, et al. Achieving tight glycemic control in the operating room: lessons learned from 12 years in the trenches of a paradigm shift in anesthetic care. Semin Thorac Cardiovasc Surg. 2006;18(4):339–45. PMID: 17395031.
83. Van den Berghe G, Wouters P, Weekers F, et al. Intensive insulin therapy in the critically ill patients. N Engl J Med. 2001;345:1359–67.

84. The hyperglycaemic response to different types of surgery and anaestheSIA. Br J Anaesth. 1970;42(1):45–53. National Diabetes Statistics Report 2020: estimates of Diabetes and its burden in the United States. 2020. https://www.cdc.gov/diabetes/data/statistics report/index.html.
85. Versteyhe S, Blanquart C, Hampe C, Mahmood S, Christoff N, De Meyts P, Gray SG, Issad T. IRS-5 and -6 are poor substrates for the insulin receptor. Mol Med Rep. 2010;3:189–93.
86. Bahadoran Z, et al. Hyperuricemia-induced endothelial insulin resistance: the nitric oxide connection. Pflügers Arch. 2022;474(Pt 3). https://doi.org/10.1007/s00424-021-02606-2.

Optimizing Postoperative Fluid and Electrolyte Care in Cardiac Surgery Patients

Khaled J. Zaza, Eynas Omer Ibrahim Abdalla, and Muhammad Firas Alhammad

Chapter Outline

1. Understand Physiological Changes: Comprehend the alterations in body fluid distribution, electrolyte concentrations, and acid–base balance that occur following cardiac surgery.
2. Identify Common Imbalances: Recognize typical postoperative fluid and electrolyte disturbances, such as hypokalemia, hyponatremia, and fluid overload.
3. Implement Management Strategies: evidence-based approaches for restoring imbalances, including the appropriate selection of fluids and electrolyte supplementation.
4. Apply Goal-Directed Therapy: Explore the principles of goal-directed fluid therapy to tailor interventions to the individual needs of each patient.
5. Prevent Complications: Understand the potential complications that can arise from improper management, including arrhythmias, renal dysfunction, and hemodynamic instability.

1 Introduction

Fluid and electrolyte management following cardiac surgery is essential for patient recovery and the prevention of perioperative complications. Cardiac surgeries often lead to significant disruptions in fluid balance and electrolyte homeostasis, which, if not properly managed, can result in adverse clinical outcomes [1]. The critical role of maintaining fluid and electrolyte balance lies in supporting hemodynamic

K. J. Zaza (✉) · E. O. I. Abdalla · M. F. Alhammad
Anaesthesia, ICU and Perioperative Medicine Department, Hamad Medical Corporation, Doha, Qatar
e-mail: kzaza@hamad.qa; eabdalla1@hamad.qa; malhammad1@hamad.qa

E. Elmistekawy, N. A. Shallik (eds.), *Perioperative Care of Cardiac Surgery Patients*, https://doi.org/10.1007/978-3-032-09817-7_9

stability, as patients undergoing cardiac surgery frequently experience shifts in intravascular and extravascular fluid compartments due to cardiopulmonary bypass (CPB) and the stress of surgery [2]. Moreover, maintaining optimal intravascular volume is crucial for ensuring adequate cardiac output, blood pressure, and organ perfusion [3].

Fluid therapy plays a crucial role in perioperative management, particularly following open-heart surgery. The surgical procedure triggers an inflammatory response, which increases vascular permeability, reduces intravascular colloid oncotic pressure, and leads to stromal edema due to diminished lymphatic flow. In the context of cardiovascular surgery involving cardiopulmonary bypass, factors such as hemodilution, hypothermia, and systemic inflammatory reactions further exacerbate vascular permeability and decrease colloid osmotic pressure, contributing to the development of interstitial edema [2, 3]. As a result, effective fluid and volume management becomes a key component in the care of patients following cardiovascular surgery.

Postoperative electrolyte disturbances, including hypokalemia, hypomagnesemia, and hyponatremia, are common and can increase the risk of arrhythmias, myocardial dysfunction, and delayed recovery [4]. Fluid overload is another concern, as it can lead to serious complications such as pulmonary edema, impaired gas exchange, and a prolonged need for ventilatory support [5]. Careful monitoring of fluid and electrolytes can help prevent complications such as third-spacing (fluid shifts into interstitial spaces) and capillary leak syndrome, as well as reduce the risk of postoperative acute kidney injury (AKI), which may occur due to hypoperfusion or nephrotoxic medications [5].

Proper fluid management also reduces the likelihood of oliguria and renal failure. Conversely, inadequate fluid resuscitation can result in hypotension, tissue hypoxia, and organ dysfunction. Achieving a balance in fluid administration helps avoid both hypovolemia and fluid overload [3]. Ultimately, effective fluid and electrolyte management facilitates early mobilization and promotes faster recovery [6].

The general principles for fluid and electrolyte management after cardiac surgery include the following:

- Individualized Goal-Directed Therapy (GDT): Tailoring fluid administration based on continuous hemodynamic monitoring and dynamic assessment of fluid status [1].
- Regular Electrolyte Monitoring: Frequent assessment of key electrolytes such as potassium, magnesium, sodium, and calcium [4].
- Balanced Crystalloids Over Colloids: Using balanced solutions like Lactated Ringer's or Plasma-Lyte may reduce complications when compared to colloid solutions.
- Diuretic Use for Fluid Overload: Carefully controlled use of diuretics, such as furosemide, to manage fluid mobilization when indicated [3].

Intravenous (IV) fluid administration is a fundamental aspect of care for all patients undergoing cardiac surgery. As such, it is essential for healthcare providers managing these patients to possess a thorough understanding of the underlying physiology and pharmacology of IV fluids. These principles influence both the pharmacodynamics of fluids (since fluids can be considered drugs) and the volume kinetics, or how patient and surgical factors affect fluid distribution and metabolism. Achieving optimal outcomes, including shorter ICU and hospital stays, reduced morbidity, and improved long-term quality of life, relies on meticulous planning, which begins in the preoperative period and continues through the intraoperative and postoperative phases [1].

An ideal fluid management strategy should aim to avoid both hypovolemia and hypervolemia, utilizing the appropriate combination of fluids administered at the optimal times. Although intravenous crystalloids and colloids are commonly used for resuscitation, they have traditionally been regarded as homogenous categories. However, the ongoing debate between crystalloids and colloids has often lacked focus. Notably, significant differences exist within these groups, such as between balanced crystalloids and saline, or starch solutions versus albumin. These variations suggest that each class of fluid should be considered separately. Despite these distinctions, large-scale international surveys indicate that the choice of fluids is more influenced by the care setting than by specific procedural or patient-related factors [2]. Appropriate fluid management post-cardiac surgery has been shown to reduce postoperative complications, thereby shortening ICU and hospital stays and lowering overall healthcare costs [1, 6].

2 Overview of Potential Complications Arising from Fluid and Electrolyte Imbalances Following Cardiac Surgery

Fluid and electrolyte imbalances are common after cardiac surgery due to the complex physiological changes that occur during and after the procedure. These disturbances can lead to a variety of postoperative complications, significantly impacting patient recovery and clinical outcomes. The following outlines the potential complications resulting from fluid and electrolyte imbalances post-cardiac surgery:

1. *Arrhythmias*: Electrolyte imbalances, particularly hypokalemia (low potassium) and hypomagnesemia (low magnesium), are key contributors to postoperative arrhythmias. Both potassium and magnesium are critical for maintaining myocardial cell membrane stability and proper electrical conduction:
   - Hypokalemia can prolong the QT interval, heightening the risk of atrial and ventricular arrhythmias, including life-threatening conditions like ventricular fibrillation [4]
   - Hypomagnesemia often coexists with hypokalemia, further exacerbating arrhythmic risks by promoting early after-depolarizations (EADs) and increasing susceptibility to torsades de pointes. Regular monitoring of serum potassium and magnesium levels is essential, with supplementation provided when levels fall below normal ranges (Potassium <4.0 mEq/L and Magnesium <2.0 mg/dL) [4].

2. *Hemodynamic Instability*: Both hypovolemia and fluid overload can lead to hemodynamic instability postoperatively:
   - Hypovolemia, often due to inadequate fluid resuscitation, bleeding, or capillary leak syndrome following cardiopulmonary bypass (CPB), can result in hypotension, reduced cardiac output, and poor organ perfusion [1, 3].
   - Fluid overload, frequently caused by excessive fluid administration or impaired renal function, can lead to pulmonary edema, heart failure, and an increased need for mechanical ventilation. Goal-directed fluid therapy (GDFT), incorporating dynamic markers such as stroke volume variation (SVV) and passive leg raise tests, can help optimize fluid management [1, 3].
3. *Neuromuscular Dysfunction*: Sodium imbalances, especially hyponatremia and hypernatremia, can lead to neuromuscular complications in the postoperative period:
   - Hyponatremia can cause confusion, seizures, and, if severe, cerebral edema [4]
   - Hypernatremia may lead to cellular dehydration, confusion, muscle weakness, and even coma. Careful management involves administering isotonic fluids for hyponatremia and providing free water replacement for hypernatremia, with gradual correction to avoid the risk of osmotic demyelination syndrome [4].
4. *Metabolic Acidosis and Alkalosis*: Metabolic imbalances such as acidosis and alkalosis can arise post-surgery:
   - Metabolic acidosis is often a result of lactic acid buildup due to tissue hypoperfusion during surgery, leading to myocardial depression and vasodilation [3, 4].
   - Metabolic alkalosis is typically caused by excessive bicarbonate administration or loss of acidic gastric contents, potentially impairing oxygen delivery by shifting the oxygen–hemoglobin dissociation curve. Identifying the underlying cause is essential, and bicarbonate use should be restricted to cases of severe metabolic acidosis (pH <7.2) [4].
5. *Renal Dysfunction (Acute Kidney Injury—AKI)*: Fluid and electrolyte imbalances can have a profound effect on renal function post-cardiac surgery, leading to acute kidney injury (AKI):
   - Electrolyte disturbances in AKI: Hyperkalemia, hyponatremia, and metabolic acidosis are common [5].
   - Causes of AKI: Prolonged CPB time, nephrotoxic drugs, and systemic inflammation contribute to the development of renal dysfunction. Early detection through regular monitoring of urine output and serum creatinine levels is crucial, along with nephroprotective strategies such as avoiding nephrotoxic medications and ensuring adequate hydration [5].
6. *Respiratory Complications*: Fluid overload can lead to pulmonary edema, impairing gas exchange and increasing the need for mechanical ventilation. Additionally, electrolyte imbalances, such as hypophosphatemia, can impact respiratory muscle function, potentially leading to respiratory failure:

- Pulmonary edema is typically caused by fluid overload or left ventricular dysfunction, leading to symptoms such as dyspnea and hypoxia [1, 3].
- Hypophosphatemia can impair diaphragmatic contractility, complicating the weaning process from mechanical ventilation [4].

3 Physiological Principles of Fluid and Electrolyte Homeostasis

- Overview of normal fluid and electrolyte distribution in the body

The human body maintains a delicate balance of fluids and electrolytes essential for normal cellular function, tissue perfusion, and overall homeostasis. Proper fluid and electrolyte distribution is critical for maintaining cellular integrity, nerve transmission, muscle contraction, and acid–base balance.

Total Body Water (TBW):

- Percentage of Body Weight:

TBW constitutes approximately 60% of total body weight in adult males and 50–55% in females due to higher fat content. In neonates, TBW can be as high as 70–75% due to lower fat content.

- Fluid Compartments:
  1. Intracellular Fluid (ICF):
     - Approx. 40% of body weight (28 liters).
     - Contains fluid inside cells.
     - Major electrolytes: Potassium (K^+) and Phosphate (PO_4^{3-}).
  2. Extracellular Fluid (ECF):
     - Approx. 20% of body weight (14 liters).
     - Further divided into:
       – Interstitial fluid (75% of ECF): Surrounds cells (10.5 liters).
       – Plasma (25% of ECF): Circulates in the vascular system (3.5 liters).
     - Major electrolytes: Sodium (Na^+) and chloride (Cl^-).

Electrolyte Composition by Compartments:

Electrolyte	Intracellular (ICF)	Extracellular (ECF)
Sodium (Na^+)	10–15 mEq/L	135–145 mEq/L
Potassium (K^+)	140–150 mEq/L	3.5–5.0 mEq/L
Calcium (Ca^{2+})	<1 mEq/L	8.5–10.5 mg/dL
Chloride (Cl^-)	3–4 mEq/L	98–106 mEq/L
Bicarbonate (HCO_3^-)	10–15 mEq/L	22–28 mEq/L
Phosphate (PO_4^{3-})	100 mEq/L	2.5–4.5 mg/dL

Electrolyte Functions

- Sodium (Na^+): A major ECF cation that plays a critical role in maintaining fluid balance, nerve function, and muscle contraction [1].
- Potassium (K^+): A major ICF cation that regulates cellular excitability and muscle contraction, particularly important in cardiac function [4].
- Calcium (Ca^{2+}): Essential for bone health, blood clotting, and neuromuscular function, also playing a significant role in cardiovascular health and cellular operations [6].
- Chloride (Cl^-): A major ECF anion, crucial for maintaining osmotic balance and acid–base homeostasis [6].
- Phosphate (PO_4^{3-}): A major ICF anion, vital for ATP production and overall cellular energy metabolism [6].
- Magnesium (Mg^{2+}): Involved in enzyme activation, muscle contraction, and nerve conduction, and plays a key role in cardiovascular and neuromuscular function [4].

Fluid Movement and Regulation

- Fluid movement between compartments is governed by osmosis, diffusion, and active transport, mechanisms driven by differences in osmotic pressure and hydrostatic pressure:

  1. Osmosis: The movement of water across membranes from areas of low solute concentration to areas of high solute concentration to equalize concentrations on both sides of the membrane.
  2. Diffusion: Movement of solutes from areas of high concentration to areas of low concentration across a permeable membrane.
  3. Active Transport: Sodium-potassium pumps actively move sodium (Na^+) out of and potassium (K^+) into cells, critical for maintaining cellular homeostasis and function [6].

Homeostatic Mechanisms Regulating Fluid Balance

- Antidiuretic Hormone (ADH): Regulates water reabsorption in the kidneys, crucial for controlling the water balance in the body, thereby affecting blood pressure and overall fluid balance [6].
- Renin-Angiotensin-Aldosterone System (RAAS): Regulates sodium retention and blood pressure, playing a critical role in fluid balance and cardiovascular stability [3].
- Atrial Natriuretic Peptide (ANP): Promotes sodium excretion in response to volume overload, helping to adjust blood volume and pressure, particularly important in postoperative settings where fluid balance can be disrupted [6].

4 Key Electrolytes and Their Roles in Cardiovascular Function

Electrolytes are fundamental in maintaining cardiovascular health, as they regulate myocardial contractility, nerve conduction, and fluid balance. The key electrolytes involved in cardiovascular function include sodium, potassium, calcium, and magnesium:

1. *Sodium (Na^+)*:
   - Sodium is crucial for maintaining extracellular fluid volume and osmotic balance.
   - It plays a key role in generating action potentials in cardiac cells through the sodium-potassium pump.
   - Imbalances such as hypernatremia or hyponatremia can result in arrhythmias and disrupted blood pressure regulation [4].
2. *Potassium (K^+)*:
   - Potassium is essential for repolarization during the cardiac action potential.
   - It helps sustain the resting membrane potential and ensures proper electrical conduction in the heart.
   - Hypokalemia (low potassium) can lead to arrhythmias, such as ventricular tachycardia, while hyperkalemia (high potassium) can cause life-threatening conditions, including cardiac arrest [4, 6].
3. *Calcium (Ca^{2+})*:
   - Calcium is vital for myocardial contraction and excitation–contraction coupling.
   - It enters cardiac cells during depolarization, triggering muscle contraction by interacting with troponin and tropomyosin.
   - Hypocalcemia can reduce cardiac contractility, whereas hypercalcemia can shorten the QT interval and increase the risk of arrhythmias [6].
4. *Magnesium (Mg^{2+})*:
   - Magnesium acts as a cofactor in numerous enzymatic reactions and is essential for ATP production.
   - It regulates calcium and potassium ion channels, helping to stabilize cardiac cell membranes.
   - Hypomagnesemia is associated with arrhythmias like torsades de pointes, while hypermagnesemia can depress myocardial excitability [4].

5 Mechanisms of Homeostasis and Factors Affecting Balance Post-Surgery

Cardiac surgery places significant stress, activating multiple systems involved in maintaining homeostasis. Understanding these mechanisms is critical for managing postoperative care and preventing complications:

1. *Neurohormonal Activation*:
   - *Sympathetic Nervous System (SNS)*: Surgery activates the SNS, leading to an increase in catecholamines (e.g., epinephrine, norepinephrine), which help regulate heart rate, blood pressure, and vascular tone, ensuring adequate tissue perfusion [1, 6].
   - *Renin-Angiotensin-Aldosterone System (RAAS)*: Blood loss and reduced renal perfusion stimulate RAAS. Angiotensin II causes vasoconstriction, while aldosterone promotes sodium and water reabsorption, stabilizing blood pressure and fluid volume [3].
   - *Hypothalamic-Pituitary-Adrenal Axis*: Stress triggers the release of cortisol, which promotes gluconeogenesis, anti-inflammatory effects, and fluid retention [3].
2. *Fluid and Electrolyte Regulation*:
   - *Osmoreceptors and Antidiuretic Hormone (ADH)*: ADH is released in response to hypovolemia or hyperosmolality, prompting water reabsorption in the kidneys to maintain circulating blood volume [6].
   - *Natriuretic Peptides*: Atrial natriuretic peptide (ANP) and brain natriuretic peptide (BNP) are released in response to cardiac stretch, facilitating sodium excretion (natriuresis) and diuresis, thus counteracting fluid overload [6].
3. *Coagulation and Hemostasis*:
   - *Platelet Activation and Clot Formation*: Tissue injury during surgery activates platelets and the coagulation cascade to prevent excessive bleeding [2].
   - *Fibrinolysis*: Balances clot formation by breaking down fibrin clots, preventing excessive thrombosis [2].
4. *Thermoregulation*:
   - *Post-surgical hypothermia*, often caused by anesthesia and prolonged exposure, is corrected through shivering and vasoconstriction, which help restore normal body temperature [2].
5. *Immune Response*:
   - *Inflammatory Mediators*: Surgery triggers the release of cytokines (e.g., IL-6, TNF-alpha) and acute-phase proteins. While essential for wound healing, excessive inflammation can lead to complications such as systemic inflammatory response syndrome (SIRS) [2, 6].

Factors Affecting Homeostatic Balance Post-Cardiac Surgery

1. *Fluid Shifts and Imbalances*:
   - *Edema and Hypovolemia*: Cardiopulmonary bypass (CPB) can cause capillary leak syndrome, resulting in fluid shifts into the interstitial space, leading to peripheral edema and hypovolemia [5].
   - *Electrolyte Abnormalities*: Imbalances such as hypokalemia (due to diuretics or RAAS activation) and hyponatremia (due to ADH overactivity) are common [4].

2. *Hemodynamic Instability*:
    - *Hypotension or Hypertension*: These may arise from SNS overactivation, the use of vasopressors, or residual effects of anesthesia [1].
3. *Cardiac Function Alterations*:
    - *Reduced myocardial contractility*, resulting from ischemia, reperfusion injury, or cardioplegia during surgery, can impair cardiac output [5].
4. *Metabolic Changes*:
    - *Hyperglycemia*: Stress-induced hyperglycemia, triggered by cortisol and catecholamine release, is common and can hinder wound healing [3].
    - *Acidosis*: Lactic acidosis, resulting from hypoperfusion or inadequate oxygen delivery, may occur following surgery [3].
5. *Coagulation and Hemorrhagic Complications*:
    - *Excessive Clotting*: Prolonged immobility and inflammation increase the risk of deep vein thrombosis (DVT) and pulmonary embolism (PE) [2].
    - *Bleeding Risk*: Anticoagulant use and platelet dysfunction due to CPB can lead to postoperative bleeding [2].
6. *Infection and Inflammation*:
    - *Postoperative infections,* such as mediastinitis or sepsis, disrupt homeostasis by exacerbating inflammatory responses [5].
7. *Respiratory Challenges*:
    - *Conditions like atelectasis, pulmonary edema, or acute respiratory distress syndrome (ARDS)* can impair oxygen delivery and acid–base balance [5].
8. *Renal Impairment*:
    - *Acute kidney injury (AKI)*, often caused by hypoperfusion, nephrotoxic medications, or inflammation, is a common complication post-cardiac surgery [5].
9. *Neurological Factors*:
    - *Cognitive dysfunction*, such as delirium or post-cardiotomy syndrome, can interfere with fluid intake, mobility, and overall recovery [5].

6 Fluid Management Strategies

Fluid management in the postoperative period following cardiac surgery is a cornerstone of recovery and plays a critical role in ensuring patient stability. An effective fluid strategy can help restore circulatory volume, optimize tissue perfusion, prevent complications such as fluid overload or dehydration, and contribute to overall recovery. This section will delve into the goals of fluid therapy, types of fluids administered, and guidelines for fluid replacement, highlighting key clinical considerations and strategies.

- *Goals of fluid therapy in the postoperative period*:
  The overarching goals of postoperative fluid therapy are to maintain hemodynamic stability, optimize tissue perfusion, and support organ function during the recovery process. Specific goals include:

- *Maintenance and replacement of fluids*
- After surgery, maintaining an equilibrium between fluid intake and output is essential to prevent both dehydration and fluid overload, which are common risks in the postoperative period. Dehydration can lead to hypotension and organ hypoperfusion, while fluid overload may strain the heart and kidneys, resulting in complications such as pulmonary edema, cardiac arrhythmias, and acute kidney injury (AKI) [7]. Following cardiac surgery, blood volume may be significantly depleted due to bleeding, fluid shifts, or intraoperative blood loss. Fluid therapy is critical to restoring intravascular volume, ensuring adequate cardiac output and perfusion to vital organs, including the brain and kidneys. Significant blood loss during surgery often necessitates replenishment with blood products or colloids. For example, patients undergoing coronary artery bypass grafting (CABG) or valve surgery frequently require blood transfusions to compensate for intraoperative losses [8].
  Postoperative patients experience insensible fluid losses through processes such as evaporation, perspiration, and respiration. These losses, which may be exacerbated in the immediate postoperative period due to factors like mechanical ventilation, fever, or surgical trauma, must be accounted for to prevent dehydration. Fluid losses from the kidneys, such as diuresis or oliguria, and the gastrointestinal tract, including nasogastric drainage or vomiting, must also be replaced. Monitoring and correcting these losses is crucial for maintaining fluid balance and ensuring optimal recovery.
- *Prevention of dehydration and fluid overload*
  Fasting, bleeding, and the body's natural fluid losses during surgery can lead to dehydration, which impairs renal perfusion and increases the risk of kidney damage and worsening clinical status. To counteract this, fluid therapy must compensate for pre-existing deficits and maintain electrolyte balance to support overall recovery. In contrast, fluid overload is a significant concern, particularly in patients with conditions such as heart failure, chronic kidney disease, or those who have undergone lengthy surgeries. Excessive fluid accumulation can result in complications like pulmonary edema, peripheral edema, and hypertension. To prevent fluid overload, careful monitoring of fluid intake, urine output, and clinical signs of fluid retention—such as edema, weight gain, or distended neck veins—is essential.

Types of Fluids Administered Postoperatively

The selection of fluids to be administered depends on the patient's clinical status, comorbidities, and the nature of the surgery. There are two primary categories of fluids used in postoperative fluid therapy: *crystalloids* and *colloids*.

- *Crystalloids vs. colloids*

Crystalloids: Crystalloids are aqueous solutions of electrolytes and small molecules that can freely pass through the vascular endothelium, entering interstitial and intracellular spaces. They are widely used for fluid resuscitation and to maintain circulatory volume after surgery. Common crystalloid solutions include normal saline, lactated Ringer's, and balanced solutions like Plasma-Lyte. Normal saline (0.9% NaCl) is frequently used post-surgery but is not ideal for long-term use due to its high chloride content, which may lead to hyperchloremic metabolic acidosis and an increased risk of acute kidney injury (AKI) [9]. Its use should be carefully monitored, particularly in patients with renal dysfunction or those at risk of acidosis. Lactated Ringer's is a more balanced solution containing sodium, potassium, calcium, and lactate, which the body metabolizes into bicarbonate. This composition helps maintain a more physiologically appropriate acid–base balance and reduces the risk of metabolic acidosis compared to normal saline. Plasma-Lyte and other balanced solutions are often preferred as they more closely resemble the body's plasma in terms of electrolyte composition. With lower chloride content, these solutions are less likely to disturb acid–base balance and are particularly valuable for cardiac surgery patients already at risk of electrolyte imbalances or renal complications. Crystalloids are typically the first-line choice for volume resuscitation when rapid expansion of circulating volume is required, such as in cases of hypovolemia, post-bleeding, or routine maintenance fluid needs.

Colloids, on the other hand, contain larger molecules such as albumin or synthetic agents like hydroxyethyl starch (HES) and dextrans [10]. These larger molecules primarily remain in the vascular space due to their size, exerting oncotic pressure that helps retain fluid within the bloodstream and prevents fluid shifts into the interstitial space. Albumin is the most commonly used colloid in postoperative care, particularly for patients who experience significant blood loss or require volume expansion that crystalloids cannot achieve alone. It is especially beneficial in cases of hypoalbuminemia, which often occurs in patients undergoing cardiac surgery. Hydroxyethyl starch is a synthetic colloid sometimes used for volume expansion, but its use is controversial due to potential risks such as renal dysfunction and coagulation disturbances, and it is typically used with caution in patients with preexisting renal impairment. Colloids are generally indicated when a larger volume of fluid is required to expand the intravascular compartment without causing significant edema. They are particularly useful in acute hypovolemic states, such as severe blood loss, or in cases of low oncotic pressure due to hypoalbuminemia.

Balanced Solutions Versus Normal Saline

- *Guidelines for fluid replacement based on clinical scenarios*

Effective fluid management after cardiac surgery must be tailored to each patient's individual needs, considering their clinical condition, the type of surgery performed, and any comorbidities. For patients with hemodynamic instability, fluid therapy should focus on restoring intravascular volume to improve cardiac output and tissue perfusion. In cases of hypotension or shock, crystalloids such as normal saline or lactated Ringer's are typically administered at rates of 500–1000 mL/hour, depending on the severity of fluid loss. If hypotension persists despite crystalloid administration, colloids or blood products may be required to stabilize hemodynamic parameters. In patients with cardiogenic shock, a more cautious approach is necessary to prevent fluid overload, with close monitoring of pulmonary status and the use of diuretics if volume overload becomes evident.

Postoperative bleeding is a significant concern in cardiac procedures, often necessitating the administration of packed red blood cells (PRBCs) to restore oxygen-carrying capacity. Decisions regarding blood transfusions should be guided by hematocrit and hemoglobin levels, as well as clinical signs of hypoperfusion, such as low urine output, tachycardia, and hypotension. In cases of coagulopathy or thrombocytopenia, additional blood products such as platelets, fresh frozen plasma (FFP), and clotting factor concentrates may be required to address bleeding complications effectively.

In patients with renal impairment, particularly those with chronic kidney disease (CKD) or those at risk of acute kidney injury (AKI) following surgery, fluid management must be conservative to avoid fluid overload. Close monitoring of kidney function, including serum creatinine, blood urea nitrogen (BUN), and urine output, is essential. If diuretics such as furosemide are used to manage fluid overload, careful monitoring of electrolytes, particularly potassium and magnesium levels, is crucial to mitigate the risk of electrolyte imbalances.

For patients with congestive heart failure (CHF), fluid restriction is critical to avoid exacerbating pulmonary edema or systemic congestion. In these cases, diuretics and diligent monitoring of fluid balance are key components of effective management. By tailoring fluid strategies to the patient's specific needs and clinical condition, optimal outcomes can be achieved while minimizing complications.

7 Managing Electrolyte Imbalances

Electrolyte imbalances are common following cardiac surgery due to a combination of surgical stress, anesthesia, fluid shifts, and the use of medications. These imbalances can affect critical aspects of patient recovery, including cardiac function, nerve conduction, and muscle contraction. Therefore, careful monitoring and correction of electrolytes are essential to improving outcomes, preventing complications, and promoting a smooth recovery. In this section, we will focus on the common electrolyte disturbances encountered in the postoperative phase, their clinical implications, and management strategies.

- *Common postoperative electrolyte imbalances and their clinical implications*:

Table 1 summarizes common postoperative electrolyte imbalances, including their etiology, clinical manifestations, and management strategies. These imbalances—hyperkalemia, hypokalemia, hyponatremia, and hypernatremia—can significantly impact patient outcomes if not promptly recognized and treated. Understanding their causes, symptoms, and appropriate interventions is essential for optimizing postoperative care.

Table 1 Common postoperative electrolyte imbalances

Electrolyte Imbalance	Etiology	Clinical Manifestations	Management
Hyperkalemia	Elevated potassium (>5.0 mmol/L) due to renal insufficiency, potassium-sparing diuretics, or potassium-containing fluids. Cellular injury during surgery releasing potassium.	Arrhythmias (ventricular tachycardia, fibrillation). Muscle weakness, fatigue, paresthesia. Severe cases: cardiac arrest.	Stabilize cardiac membrane with calcium gluconate (10–20 mL of 10%). Shift potassium into cells with insulin + glucose or sodium bicarbonate if acidotic. Remove potassium using diuretics, Kayexalate, or hemodialysis.
Hypokalemia	Potassium <3.5 mmol/L from diuresis, GI losses (vomiting, diarrhea), or inadequate intake. Loop or thiazide diuretics can cause significant depletion.	Muscle weakness, cramps, fatigue, constipation. Arrhythmias (PVCs, atrial fibrillation). Severe cases: paralysis, respiratory failure, cardiac arrest.	Oral potassium supplementation if tolerable. IV potassium for severe cases, cautious infusion (<10–20 mmol/hour). Monitor serum potassium; recommend potassium-rich foods.
Hyponatremia	Sodium <135 mmol/L due to fluid overload, hypotonic fluids (5% dextrose), SIADH, or renal dysfunction.	Symptoms range from nausea, headache to severe confusion, seizures, coma, and brain herniation. Cardiac and neurological impairments.	Restrict fluid intake. Hypertonic saline (3% NaCl) for severe cases, administered slowly. Treat underlying causes (e.g., SIADH, fluid overload). Consider vasopressin antagonists if refractory.
Hypernatremia	Sodium >145 mmol/L due to inadequate fluid intake, excessive diuresis, hyperventilation, fever, or hypertonic solutions (e.g., sodium bicarbonate).	Thirst, irritability, confusion, muscle twitching. Severe cases: seizures, coma, intracellular dehydration causing neurological impairment.	Gradual fluid replacement with hypotonic solutions (0.45% saline, D5W). IV therapy if oral intake is inadequate. Monitor serum sodium to guide therapy and prevent cerebral edema.

- *Treatment strategies for correcting imbalances*:
- The treatment of electrolyte imbalances depends on the *severity*, *underlying cause*, and *patient-specific factors* such as comorbidities and response to previous treatments. For each imbalance, the management approach should be individualized.
  - *Pharmacological interventions (e.g., potassium replacement, sodium correction)*
  - Pharmacological interventions play a crucial role in managing postoperative electrolyte imbalances to ensure patient stability and prevent complications.

Potassium replacement is commonly administered either orally or intravenously, depending on the severity of hypokalemia. Oral potassium chloride is preferred for mild to moderate cases, while intravenous potassium chloride, diluted in saline, is reserved for more severe imbalances. Sodium imbalances, such as hyponatremia or hypernatremia, require careful and gradual correction to prevent severe complications like cerebral edema in hypernatremia or central pontine myelinolysis in cases of rapid hyponatremia correction. In severe hyperkalemia, calcium gluconate or calcium chloride is administered to stabilize cardiac function and mitigate the risk of life-threatening arrhythmias. Additionally, abnormalities in magnesium and phosphate levels must be addressed. Magnesium supplementation is vital for correcting hypomagnesemia, which can worsen arrhythmias, while phosphate replacement is necessary for treating hypophosphatemia, often seen in patients with prolonged fasting or malnutrition.

– *Dietary considerations and restrictions*

  Postoperative cardiac surgery patients often benefit from specific dietary recommendations to maintain electrolyte balance and support recovery. Sodium intake should be restricted, particularly for patients with heart failure or hypertension, to reduce fluid retention and prevent exacerbation of high blood pressure. For patients experiencing hypokalemia, a diet rich in potassium is encouraged, including foods like bananas, oranges, spinach, and potatoes. Additionally, patients on long-term diuretics or those with renal dysfunction may require phosphate and magnesium supplementation, which can be achieved through dietary sources or pharmacological means to address deficiencies and support overall electrolyte stability.

- *Monitoring and adjusting electrolyte management based on patient response*

Effective electrolyte management requires regular monitoring of serum levels, including sodium, potassium, calcium, magnesium, and phosphorus, to ensure that interventions are both appropriate and effective. Therapy should be guided by the patient's clinical response, such as symptom improvement and normalization of vital signs. Adjustments to treatments, such as diuretics, should be made based on fluid balance and renal function. Additionally, urine output, ECG changes, and findings from clinical examinations should be carefully evaluated to inform and optimize electrolyte therapy.

- *Special Considerations in Fluid and Electrolyte Management*

In the postoperative phase of cardiac surgery, managing fluid and electrolyte balance becomes even more complex due to a variety of patient-specific factors, including pre-existing comorbidities, medications, and the nature of the surgery. These special considerations require a nuanced approach, with individualized fluid and electrolyte strategies tailored to optimize recovery and prevent complications. This section discusses key factors that influence fluid and electrolyte management in this population, including the presence of comorbidities such as *renal failure* and *heart failure*, the impact of medications, and the role of patient characteristics (e.g., age, weight, preoperative fluid status).

- *Managing patients with comorbidities (e.g., renal failure, heart failure)*

Failure Acute Kidney Injury (AKI) is a common complication following cardiac surgery, particularly in patients with pre-existing kidney disease, intraoperative hypotension, nephrotoxic medications, or prolonged surgery. Fluid and electrolyte management in these patients can be challenging due to their compromised ability to excrete excess fluids and regulate electrolytes. Fluid overload is a significant risk in AKI, potentially leading to pulmonary edema, cardiogenic shock, and worsening renal function. Careful monitoring of fluid balance, urine output, and renal function is crucial. Fluid resuscitation should be cautious, with balanced crystalloids preferred, and excessive IV fluids should be avoided. In some cases, diuretics, such as furosemide, may be used to maintain fluid balance, but their use should be closely monitored. Common electrolyte disturbances in AKI include hyperkalemia, hyperphosphatemia, and hypocalcemia. Potassium levels should be monitored frequently, and in cases of hyperkalemia, immediate interventions like calcium gluconate, insulin with glucose, or sodium bicarbonate may be necessary. Phosphate binders and magnesium levels should also be carefully managed, as the kidneys play a key role in excreting these electrolytes. In severe cases, dialysis may be required to manage fluid overload and correct electrolyte imbalances.

Patients with pre-existing chronic kidney disease (CKD) require close monitoring, especially in the immediate postoperative period. The goal is to prevent further deterioration of kidney function while managing fluid balance. Many CKD patients are at risk of fluid overload, and fluid intake may need to be restricted. Daily weight, urine output, and serum creatinine levels should be carefully monitored. These patients may also have chronic electrolyte abnormalities, such as hyperkalemia and hyperphosphatemia, which require regular monitoring and, if necessary, adjustment of medications like potassium or phosphate binders.

In patients with heart failure, particularly those with congestive heart failure (CHF), fluid overload is a concern due to the compromised ability of the heart to handle fluid volume [11]. Fluid retention can lead to pulmonary edema, peripheral edema, hypertension, and worsening heart failure symptoms. A conservative approach to fluid administration is often necessary, with fluid intake restricted and daily fluid balance closely monitored. The target is to maintain a negative fluid balance, meaning fluid output should exceed intake, to prevent fluid retention. Loop diuretics, such as furosemide, are commonly used to promote fluid removal and relieve symptoms of congestion, such as shortness of breath and peripheral edema. However, careful monitoring is required to avoid electrolyte disturbances, such as hypokalemia and hyponatremia, and renal dysfunction. Sodium intake should also be limited to 2–3 grams per day to help prevent fluid retention and worsening symptoms.

Cardiac surgery often results in stress hyperglycemia, especially in patients with pre-existing diabetes mellitus. Elevated glucose levels can impair wound healing, increase the risk of infections, and exacerbate fluid and electrolyte imbalances. Tight glucose control is recommended in the postoperative period, often using intravenous insulin drips to maintain blood glucose levels within a target range. Continuous glucose monitoring (CGM) or frequent blood glucose testing should guide insulin therapy [12]. Patients should be monitored for hypokalemia, as insulin therapy can shift potassium into cells. High glucose levels can lead to hyperosmolarity and affect fluid shifts, contributing to dehydration and electrolyte disturbances like hypokalemia and hyponatremia. Rehydration with appropriate IV fluids and correction of electrolyte imbalances are critical to managing these patients effectively.

- *Individualized fluid and electrolyte strategies based on patient characteristics (age, weight, prior fluid status)*

Older adults are particularly vulnerable to both fluid dehydration and fluid overload due to age-related physiological changes, including reduced renal function, lower muscle mass (which affects fluid volume), and altered thirst mechanisms. Their renal clearance is often diminished, making it harder to excrete excess fluids or correct electrolyte imbalances. For these patients, more cautious and conservative fluid management is necessary. Close monitoring of renal function, including serum creatinine levels, urine output, and daily weight, is essential. Frequent reassessment is needed to avoid fluid overload, as older adults are at higher risk due to these physiological changes. Additionally, older adults are more susceptible to electrolyte imbalances, such as hyponatremia, hypokalemia, and hyperkalemia, especially when taking medications like diuretics, antihypertensives, and antiarrhythmic agents. These patients often require more frequent monitoring and individualized adjustments in electrolyte therapy.

Obese patients undergoing cardiac surgery present unique challenges for fluid and electrolyte management because of changes in body fluid compartments. Obese individuals tend to have higher extracellular fluid volumes and may require adjustments in fluid resuscitation to avoid both under-resuscitation and over-resuscitation [13]. The obese population is at greater risk for fluid overload after surgery, requiring close monitoring and individualized fluid therapy. In these patients, fluid administration should be based on ideal body weight rather than total body weight to avoid excessive volume resuscitation. Additionally, obese patients may be at risk for hyperkalemia if they have associated renal dysfunction or are taking potassium-sparing medications.

Patients with significant preoperative dehydration are at risk for hypovolemia and electrolyte imbalances. This dehydration may be caused by inadequate fluid intake, bleeding, or prolonged fasting, and can compromise renal perfusion, making fluid resuscitation more difficult in the postoperative period. Preoperative dehydration can lead to difficulties in maintaining fluid balance during and after surgery. Therefore, preoperative fluid status should be assessed and corrected as much as possible before surgery. In cases of dehydration, volume resuscitation may need to be more aggressive in the immediate postoperative period to restore circulating volume and prevent complications like acute kidney injury and hypotension. Dehydrated patients may have elevated sodium levels (hypernatremia), especially if they were unable to maintain adequate oral intake before surgery. Gradual fluid replacement using hypotonic solutions, such as 0.45% NaCl, is recommended to carefully correct the electrolyte imbalances and restore proper fluid balance.

- *Implications of medications on fluid and electrolyte balance (e.g., diuretics, anticoagulants)*

Medications play a significant role in the postoperative management of fluid and electrolytes, as many drugs commonly used during the perioperative period can directly affect fluid balance and electrolyte levels. Diuretics, commonly used in patients with heart failure, renal insufficiency, or pulmonary edema, can lead to fluid loss and electrolyte imbalances, such as hypokalemia, hyponatremia, and hypomagnesemia. Close monitoring of serum electrolytes and renal function is required for patients on diuretics to prevent complications. Potassium supplementation may be necessary if hypokalemia develops.

Anticoagulants, such as heparin, warfarin, and newer oral anticoagulants (NOACs), can influence fluid balance indirectly by increasing the risk of bleeding, which can lead to hypovolemia and hemodynamic instability. Careful monitoring is essential for patients on anticoagulants, and appropriate interventions should be initiated if excessive blood loss occurs, such as blood transfusions or the use of reversal agents.

Vasopressors and inotropes, such as norepinephrine and dopamine, are often used in critically ill postoperative patients to support blood pressure and cardiac output. While these drugs are vital for hemodynamic support, they can also cause electrolyte shifts. Vasopressors can induce vasoconstriction, reducing blood flow to organs, including the kidneys, which may impact renal function and contribute to electrolyte imbalances, such as hyperkalemia.

8 Case Studies

8.1 Case 1: Fluid Overload in a Post-Cardiac Surgery Patient with Heart Failure

A 72-year-old patient with a history of congestive heart failure (CHF), diabetes mellitus, and hypertension underwent coronary artery bypass grafting (CABG). On postoperative day 2, the patient presented with shortness of breath, orthopnea, and bilateral lower extremity edema. Vital signs showed a blood pressure of 160/95 mmHg, heart rate of 92 bpm, and respiratory rate of 22 breaths/min. There was noticeable jugular venous distention (JVD), and auscultation revealed crackles in both lungs. The patient's fluid status was concerning for fluid overload, likely exacerbated by compromised cardiac output and postoperative fluid administration.

Initial bloodwork revealed normal sodium levels but mild hypokalemia ($K+ = 3.3$ mmol/L) and elevated B-type natriuretic peptide (BNP) levels, indicative of a heart failure exacerbation. Serum creatinine was slightly elevated (1.4 mg/dL, baseline 1.2 mg/dL), suggesting renal stress due to fluid overload. Management focused on fluid restriction, with total daily intake limited to 1.5 liters and unnecessary intravenous fluid expansion eliminated. A high-dose loop diuretic (furosemide, 40 mg IV bolus) was given to promote fluid excretion, with diuretic therapy adjusted according to urine output to achieve negative fluid balance. The patient's hypokalemia was addressed with oral potassium supplementation and close monitoring of serum potassium and magnesium levels.

Continuous monitoring of vital signs, fluid balance, urine output, and electrocardiogram (ECG) for arrhythmias was essential. By postoperative day 4, the patient's symptoms of fluid overload improved significantly. Shortness of breath and edema resolved, urine output increased to 2.5 liters per day, and diuretics were gradually tapered down. Electrolytes, including potassium, were repleted and stabilized. The patient was discharged on oral diuretics with instructions for monitoring fluid intake and potassium levels.

Key learning points include the importance of cautious fluid management and early diuretic therapy in cardiac surgery patients with a history of heart failure to prevent complications. Frequent monitoring and correction of electrolytes, particularly potassium and magnesium, is critical, as diuretics can induce significant disturbances. Close attention to renal function and fluid status is crucial for preventing further complications, particularly in elderly patients with comorbidities like CHF.

8.2 Case 2: Hyponatremia in a Post-CABG Patient with Renal Impairment

A 68-year-old patient with chronic kidney disease (CKD), hypertension, and hyperlipidemia underwent coronary artery bypass grafting (CABG). On postoperative day 3, the patient developed confusion, lethargy, and nausea. Vital signs included a blood pressure of 130/75 mmHg and a heart rate of 85 bpm. The patient was oliguric, producing only 300 mL of urine over 24 hours, with decreased skin turgor and dry mucous membranes. Mental status changes raised concerns for a possible electrolyte disturbance.

Laboratory tests revealed serum sodium of 128 mmol/L, indicating hyponatremia. The patient's urine sodium concentration was low (<10 mmol/L), suggesting that the kidneys were conserving sodium due to perceived dehydration or inadequate fluid intake. Serum creatinine had increased to 2.2 mg/dL (baseline 1.4 mg/dL), indicating worsening renal function. The patient's fluid status appeared to be compromised, likely due to inadequate oral intake, increased fluid loss, and the effects of surgery. A component of Syndrome of Inappropriate Antidiuretic Hormone Secretion (SIADH) was also considered as a contributing factor to the hyponatremia.

Management began with the administration of normal saline to re-expand intravascular volume and address hypovolemia. Sodium levels were corrected cautiously using hypertonic saline (3% NaCl) at a slow infusion rate of 100 mL per hour. Sodium levels were closely monitored, with the goal of increasing them by no more than 6 mmol/L per day. Diuretics were withheld to prevent further fluid depletion, and kidney function was closely monitored. Diuretic therapy would be resumed only after renal function recovered and fluid balance improved. Given the possibility of SIADH, urine and serum osmolality were monitored to guide treatment. After 48 hours of careful fluid and sodium management, the patient's mental status improved, and serum sodium gradually increased to 132 mmol/L. Urine output increased, and renal function showed signs of recovery, with serum creatinine returning to baseline levels. The patient was transferred to the general ward and discharged with follow-up nephrology care for ongoing monitoring of kidney function. Key learning points include the common occurrence of hyponatremia in postoperative patients, especially those with renal dysfunction or those receiving large volumes of hypotonic fluids. Fluid resuscitation should be approached cautiously to correct both hypovolemia and hyponatremia, avoiding rapid sodium correction, which can result in central pontine myelinolysis. In patients with chronic kidney disease, close attention to renal function and electrolyte balance is essential due to their impaired ability to manage fluid shifts and electrolyte disturbances.

8.3 Case 3: Hyperkalemia in a Post-Cardiac Surgery Patient on Diuretics

A 56-year-old patient with hypertension, type 2 diabetes, and coronary artery disease (CAD) underwent mitral valve replacement. On postoperative day 1, the patient developed lethargy, muscle weakness, and an abnormal heart rhythm. An ECG revealed peaked T waves and widened QRS complexes, suggestive of hyperkalemia. Laboratory tests confirmed a serum potassium level of 6.5 mmol/L, indicating hyperkalemia. Renal function was normal, with a serum creatinine of 1.1 mg/dL, indicating no significant renal impairment. A medication review showed that the patient had been prescribed high-dose loop diuretics postoperatively for fluid management. Additionally, the patient had been on potassium-sparing diuretics (e.g., spironolactone) prior to surgery, which could have contributed to potassium retention.

Management included immediate treatment to stabilize the cardiac membrane with an intravenous calcium gluconate infusion. A bicarbonate infusion was also administered to shift potassium into cells. The patient was given a potassium binder (e.g., sodium polystyrene sulfonate) and instructed to discontinue potassium-sparing diuretics. Loop diuretics were continued, with close monitoring of serum electrolytes to prevent further potassium loss. If potassium levels did not improve, hemodialysis was considered. After 12 hours of treatment, the patient's potassium level decreased to 5.2 mmol/L, and the ECG returned to normal. Symptoms of muscle weakness and lethargy improved significantly. The potassium binder was discontinued, and potassium supplementation was carefully adjusted to maintain normal levels.

Key learning points include that hyperkalemia is a life-threatening postoperative complication, especially in patients on potassium-sparing diuretics or medications like ACE inhibitors and ARBs. Early identification and treatment with calcium gluconate, bicarbonate, and insulin are essential to manage severe hyperkalemia and prevent arrhythmias. Patients on diuretics require careful and continuous monitoring of electrolytes to avoid both hyperkalemia and hypokalemia.

9 Managing Fluid and Electrolyte Imbalances Post Cardiac Surgery

- *Complications Associated with Fluid and Electrolyte Imbalances*

Fluid and electrolyte imbalances post cardiac surgery are common and potentially life-threatening complications, often resulting from the complex interplay of surgical stress, cardiopulmonary bypass (CPB), and pre-existing comorbidities.

These imbalances can lead to conditions such as cardiac surgery-associated acute kidney injury (CSA-AKI), fluid overload, and postoperative atrial fibrillation (POAF). CSA-AKI, has an incidence of 20–40%, is associated with increased morbidity, mortality, and prolonged hospital stays [14, 15]. Fluid overload may contribute to pulmonary edema, cardiac dysfunction, and prolonged mechanical ventilation, while hypovolemia, may result in decreased tissue perfusion and organ failure [14, 16].

Electrolyte disturbances, particularly in sodium, potassium, and calcium levels, further complicate recovery. For example, hyperkalemia or hypokalemia can precipitate life-threatening arrhythmias, while hyponatremia is associated with neurological symptoms, including seizures and encephalopathy [1, 2].

In CPB, hemodilution, inflammatory activation, and increased capillary permeability contribute significantly to fluid shifts and interstitial edema. Disruption of the endothelial glycocalyx, a key regulator of vascular permeability, has been implicated as a central mechanism. The degradation of glycocalyx components, such as syndecan-1 and heparan sulfate, due to ischemia-reperfusion injury, inflammation, and fluid overload, exacerbates tissue edema and organ dysfunction [2, 14]. POAF, a complication in up to 50% of coronary artery bypass grafting (CABG) patients, has also been correlated with fluid imbalances on the day of surgery, emphasizing the need for targeted fluid management strategies [2, 15, 17].

- *Strategies to Address Fluid and Electrolyte Imbalances*
  Effective management of fluid and electrolyte imbalances post cardiac surgery requires a multimodal approach encompassing precise monitoring, evidence-based interventions, and individualized therapy. The following strategies have been identified as critical for optimizing outcomes:

1. *Individualized Fluid Management*
   Tailoring fluid therapy based on patient-specific factors, including baseline volume status, type of surgery, and intraoperative fluid shifts, is essential. Dynamic indices such as stroke volume variation and pulse pressure variation should guide fluid resuscitation to prevent both hypovolemia and fluid overload [2, 18]. The Perioperative Quality Initiative (POQI) emphasizes individualized perioperative fluid management to account for patient comorbidities and surgical complexity [1].
2. *Optimizing Electrolyte Balance*
   Close monitoring of serum electrolytes, especially potassium, magnesium, calcium, and sodium, is critical. Hypokalemia and hyperkalemia must be corrected promptly using balanced potassium supplementation protocols. Hypocalcemia, a common issue following CPB, should be addressed with calcium gluconate or chloride as needed. Regular arterial blood gas analysis can guide the correction of acid–base disturbances [14, 16].
3. *Balanced Crystalloids and Colloids*
   Balanced crystalloids, such as lactated Ringer's or Plasma-Lyte, are preferred over normal saline to minimize complications such as hyperchloremic acidosis and their adverse effects on renal function. Colloids, such as albumin, may be utilized in selected patients with significant hypoalbuminemia to restore oncotic pressure, but their use should be judicious to minimize the risk of capillary leak and interstitial edema [19, 20].
4. *Prevention of Endothelial Glycocalyx Damage*
   Protecting the glycocalyx is pivotal in preventing excessive capillary leakage and tissue edema. Strategies include limiting pump time and biocompatible circuitry, avoiding excessive fluid loading, and using anti-inflammatory agents to reduce cytokine-mediated glycocalyx degradation [2]. Emerging therapies such as hydrocortisone, vitamin C, and thiamine may offer additional protective effects.
5. *Targeted Diuretic Therapy*
   Postoperative fluid overload is often managed with diuretics. Loop diuretics, such as furosemide, are first-line agents, but they may cause electrolyte depletion. Tolvaptan, a selective vasopressin V2 receptor antagonist, has shown promise in managing fluid overload by promoting aquaresis without significant electrolyte loss. Its use is particularly advantageous in patients with renal impairment or refractory fluid overload [16, 18].
6. *Integration of Hemodynamic Monitoring*
   Advanced hemodynamic monitoring tools, including transpulmonary thermodilution and transesophageal echocardiography (TEE), provide critical insights into fluid responsiveness and cardiac function. These technologies enable precise titration of fluids, vasopressors, and inotropes [14, 16].

7. *Postoperative Protocols for Fluid Stewardship*
   Postoperative care should emphasize fluid stewardship, including early mobilization and minimization of unnecessary fluid administration. The concept of "de-resuscitation" involves the careful removal of excess fluids through diuretics or ultrafiltration in patients with ongoing fluid overload [1, 18].

10 Future Directions and Research

Opportunities to bridge significant gaps in knowledge and develop advancements in perioperative care post cardiac surgery exist. Future research may focus on:

- *Biomarker Development*: As identifying biomarkers for early detection of CSA-AKI, fluid overload, and electrolyte imbalances enable preemptive interventions [15, 19, 21].
- *Precision Medicine in Fluid and Electrolyte Management*
- Personalized protocols considering genetic predispositions, preoperative conditions, and surgical risk profiles may offer better fluid optimization and electrolyte care in cardiac surgery [14, 19].
- *Emerging Therapies*
- The efficacy and long-term outcomes of endothelial glycocalyx-protective agents and novel diuretics like tolvaptan should be evaluated in cardiac surgery patients through larger multicenter trials [2, 21, 22].
- *Artificial Intelligence (AI) in Fluid Management*

- AI-driven decision support systems may analyze and integrate real-time data to recommend fluid adjustments, anticipate complications like CSA-AKI or POAF, and optimize patient outcomes [1].

11 Chapter Summary Points

1. *Importance of Fluid and Electrolyte Management*: Proper management of fluids and electrolytes is vital for patient recovery and preventing complications after cardiac surgery, as surgeries can significantly disrupt fluid balance and electrolyte homeostasis.
2. *Fluid Dynamics in Surgery*: Cardiopulmonary bypass (CPB) and surgical stress lead to shifts in fluid compartments, exacerbating vascular permeability and reducing colloid osmotic pressure. This necessitates careful fluid and volume management to prevent interstitial edema and other related complications.
3. *Complications from Electrolyte Imbalances*: Postoperative conditions like hypokalemia, hypomagnesemia, and hyponatremia increase the risk of arrhythmias and myocardial dysfunction. Managing these electrolyte disturbances is critical for stabilizing patients and promoting recovery.

4. *Strategies for Fluid Administration*: Goal-directed therapy, regular monitoring of electrolytes, and the preference for balanced crystalloids over colloids mitigates complications and supports recovery.
5. *Postoperative Monitoring and Management*: Continuous monitoring of fluid and electrolyte levels postoperatively is essential to prevent severe complications like acute kidney injury and fluid overload.
6. *Overall Importance of Individualized Care*: The chapter emphasizes the need for individualized fluid and electrolyte management tailored to each patient's specific conditions and responses. This helps enhance outcomes and reduce hospital stays and healthcare costs.

References

1. Ostermann M, Auzinger G, Grocott M, Morton-Bailey V, Raphael J, Shaw AD, et al. Perioperative fluid management: evidence-based consensus recommendations from the international multidisciplinary PeriOperative Quality Initiative. Br J Anaesth. 2024;133:1263–75.
2. Nishi H. Advent of new perioperative care for fluid management after cardiovascular surgery: a review of current evidence. J Cardiol. 2020;75:606–13. https://doi.org/10.1016/j.jjcc.2019.12.010.
3. Shaw A, Raghunathan K. Fluid management in cardiac surgery: colloid or crystalloid? Anesthesiol Clin. 2013;31:269–80. https://doi.org/10.1016/j.anclin.2012.12.007.
4. Rassam SS, Counsell DJ. Perioperative electrolyte and fluid balance. Contin Educ Anaesth Crit Care Pain. 2005;5:157–60. https://doi.org/10.1093/bjaceaccp/mki042.
5. Udzik J, Sienkiewicz S, Biskupski A, Szylińska A, Kowalska Z, Biskupski P. Cardiac complications following cardiac surgery procedures. J Clin Med. 2020;9:3347. https://doi.org/10.3390/jcm9103347.
6. Martin GS, Bassett P. Crystalloids vs. colloids for fluid resuscitation in the intensive care unit: a systematic review and meta-analysis. J Crit Care. 2019;50:144–54. https://doi.org/10.1016/j.jcrc.2018.11.031.
7. Kayilioglu SI, Dinc T, Sozen I, Bostanoglu A, Cete M, Coskun F. Postoperative fluid management. World J Crit care Med. 2015;4:192–201. https://doi.org/10.5492/wjccm.v4.i3.192.
8. Arias-Morales CE, Stoicea N, Gonzalez-Zacarias AA, Slawski D, Bhandary SP, Saranteas T, et al. Revisiting blood transfusion and predictors of outcome in cardiac surgery patients: a concise perspective. F1000Res. 2017;6. https://doi.org/10.12688/f1000research.10085.1.
9. Curran JD, Major P, Tang K, Bagshaw SM, Dionne JC, Menon K, et al. Comparison of balanced crystalloid solutions: a systematic review and meta-analysis of randomized controlled trials. Crit Care Explor. 2021;3:e0398. https://doi.org/10.1097/CCE.0000000000000398.
10. Lewis SR, Pritchard MW, Evans DJ, Butler AR, Alderson P, Smith AF, et al. Colloids versus crystalloids for fluid resuscitation in critically ill people. Cochrane Database Syst Rev. 2018;8:CD000567. https://doi.org/10.1002/14651858.CD000567.pub7.
11. Wittczak A, Ślot M, Bielecka-Dabrowa A. The importance of optimal hydration in patients with heart failure—not always too much fluid. Biomedicine. 2023;11:2684. https://doi.org/10.3390/biomedicines11102684.
12. Miller EM. Using continuous glucose monitoring in clinical practice. Clin Diabetes. 2020;38:429–38. https://doi.org/10.2337/cd20-0043.
13. Rae L, Pham TN, Carrougher G, Honari S, Gibran NS, Arnoldo BD, et al. Differences in resuscitation in morbidly obese burn patients may contribute to high mortality. J Burn Care Res. 2013;34:507–14. https://doi.org/10.1097/BCR.0b013e3182a2a771.
14. Malbrain MLNG, et al. Rational use of intravenous fluids in critically ill patients. 2024.

15. Palomba H, Treml RE, Caldonazo T, Katayama HT, Gomes BC, Malbouisson LMS, et al. Intraoperative fluid balance and cardiac surgery-associated acute kidney injury: a multicenter prospective study. Braz J Anesthesiol (English Ed). 2022;72:688–94.
16. Young R. Perioperative fluid and electrolyte management in cardiac surgery: a review. J Extra Corpor Technol. 2012;44:20–6.
17. Foroughi M. Introduction and history of postoperative care for adult cardiac surgical patients. In: Postoperative critical care for adult cardiac surgical patients. Cham: Springer International Publishing; 2018. p. 1–5. https://doi.org/10.1007/978-3-319-75747-6_1.
18. Hessel EA, Groom RC. Guidelines for conduct of cardiopulmonary bypass. J Cardiothorac Vasc Anesth. 2021;35:1–17.
19. Chen X, Xu J, Li Y, Shen B, Jiang W, Luo Z, et al. The effect of postoperative fluid balance on the occurrence and progression of acute kidney injury after cardiac surgery. J Cardiothorac Vasc Anesth. 2021;35:2700–6. https://doi.org/10.1053/j.jvca.2020.10.007.
20. Dabbagh A, Esmailian F, Aranki S. Postoperative critical care for adult cardiac surgical patients. Cham: Springer International Publishing; 2018. https://doi.org/10.1007/978-3-319-75747-6.
21. Xiao Y, Zhao C, Xu J, Pan G. Fluid balance and risk of postoperative atrial fibrillation after on-pump coronary artery bypass grafting surgery. Heart Surg Forum. 2024;27:E789–96. https://doi.org/10.59958/hsf.7661.
22. Young R. Perioperative fluid and electrolyte management in cardiac surgery: a review. J Extra Corpor Technol. 2012;44:P20–6. http://www.ncbi.nlm.nih.gov/pubmed/22730868.

Postoperative Renal and Urinary Care of Cardiac Surgical Patients

Ibrahim A. Khalil, Raghad Aljariri, Vara Lakshmi Kolati, Tarlq Al Safi, and Mohannad Romeh

1 Introduction

Cardiac surgery is a significant risk factor for acute kidney injury (AKI), affecting 5–43% of patients and contributing to increased mortality, prolonged hospital stays, and substantial healthcare costs [1–9]. Even among those who regain full renal function, there remains a heightened risk of chronic kidney disease (CKD) and long-term mortality. Notably, approximately 1% of patients develop new dialysis dependence following surgery [5, 10–12].

The incidence and severity of AKI vary based on the type of cardiac surgery performed. Coronary artery bypass grafting (CABG) has the lowest reported incidence (19%), while valve surgeries (27.5%) and aortic procedures (29%) carry higher risks [13, 14]. Other key determinants of post-cardiac surgery renal failure include preoperative renal function and the duration of surgery [10].

The pathogenesis of cardiac surgery–associated AKI (CSA-AKI) is multifactorial. Hemodynamic instability, ischemia-reperfusion injury, systemic inflammation, and exposure to nephrotoxic medications all contribute to kidney injury. Additionally, the choice of cardiopulmonary bypass techniques and perioperative fluid management strategies play critical roles [15, 16].

I. A. Khalil (✉)
Department of Urology, Hamad Medical Corporation, Doha, Qatar

R. Aljariri
School of Medicine, University of Jordan, Amman, Jordan

V. L. Kolati · T. Al Safi
Anaesthesia, ICU and Perioperative Medicine Department, Hamad Medical Corporation, Doha, Qatar

M. Romeh
Life Care Hospital, Freetown, Sierra Leone

E. Elmistekawy, N. A. Shallik (eds.), *Perioperative Care of Cardiac Surgery Patients*, https://doi.org/10.1007/978-3-032-09817-7_10

Beyond AKI, urological complications are common after cardiac surgery. Urinary tract infections (UTIs), catheter-associated UTIs (CAUTIs), urinary retention, and hematuria [17].

This chapter provides a comprehensive overview of renal and urological complications following cardiac surgery, highlighting risk factors, pathophysiological mechanisms, prevention strategies, and best practices for postoperative management.

2 Cardiac Surgery–Associated AKI

2.1 Pathophysiology of CSA-AKI

CSA-AKI results from multiple interrelated mechanisms, including renal hypoperfusion, ischemia-reperfusion injury (IRI), inflammation, oxidative stress, nephrotoxin exposure, and genetic factors, occurring throughout the perioperative period.

2.1.1 Renal Hypoperfusion and Ischemia-Reperfusion Injury

The renal medulla's high metabolic demand and low oxygen tension (10–20 mmHg) make it prone to hypoxic injury [15]. CPB-associated factors such as low flow, hemodilution, emboli, rewarming, and hemolysis contribute to renal ischemia [18–21]. Prolonged ischemia leads to tubular damage, oxidative stress, and inflammation [22].

Low cardiac output and persistent hypotension activate the sympathetic nervous system and RAAS, leading to systemic vasoconstriction and reduced renal perfusion [18–23]. Venous congestion, an independent CSA-AKI risk factor, further impairs perfusion and GFR [24, 25]. Optimizing oxygen delivery during CPB has been shown to reduce CSA-AKI by 50% [26]. Reperfusion injury post-CPB triggers mitochondrial dysfunction and reactive oxygen species (ROS) production, exacerbating inflammation and renal injury [27].

2.1.2 Inflammation and Oxidative Stress

CPB-induced systemic inflammation activates endothelial cells, immune pathways, and cytokines, leading to tubular injury [28, 29]. Reperfusion of hypoxic tissue generates ROS, further driving inflammation and endothelial dysfunction [30, 31]. Hypoxia-induced endothelial damage and leukocyte adhesion worsen nitric oxide synthesis and oxygen delivery [32].

CPB-related hemolysis releases free hemoglobin and iron, catalyzing oxidative damage and lipid peroxidation [33, 34]. IRI amplifies free iron toxicity, impairing renal epithelial cells and promoting oxidative stress–mediated tissue damage [35].

2.1.3 Nephrotoxin-Induced Injury

Common perioperative nephrotoxins include NSAIDs, ACE inhibitors (ACEis), ARBs, aminoglycosides, diuretics, and contrast agents. NSAIDs exacerbate medullary hypoxia, while ACEis and ARBs impair renal hemodynamics [15, 36, 37]. Aminoglycosides have dose-dependent nephrotoxicity [38], and prophylactic diuretics like furosemide have no proven benefit in AKI prevention [39]. High-dose contrast agents before surgery elevate AKI risk [40].

2.1.4 Metabolic and Neurohormonal Activation

Cardiac surgery activates the sympathetic nervous system and the hypothalamic-pituitary-adrenal axis, increasing vasopressin, catecholamines, and endothelin-1, leading to vasoconstriction and renal hypoperfusion [41, 42]. CPB-induced hemolysis releases free iron, driving oxidative stress and vasoconstriction [43]. Hepcidin regulates iron homeostasis, reducing IRI-induced tubular damage and inflammation [44]. Iron chelation therapy is being explored as an AKI prevention strategy [45].

2.1.5 Genetic Susceptibility to CSA-AKI

Genetic polymorphisms in angiotensinogen, APOE, ACE, eNOS, IL-6, IL-10, STAT3, and MIF genes influence CSA-AKI risk, though findings remain inconsistent [46–48]. Understanding genetic predispositions may refine risk stratification and patient management.

Figure 1 summarizes key contributors to renal dysfunction during and after cardiopulmonary bypass, including hypotension, microvascular inflammation, fibrin deposition, and CPB-induced shear forces, which impair renal perfusion and filtration, potentially causing acute kidney injury

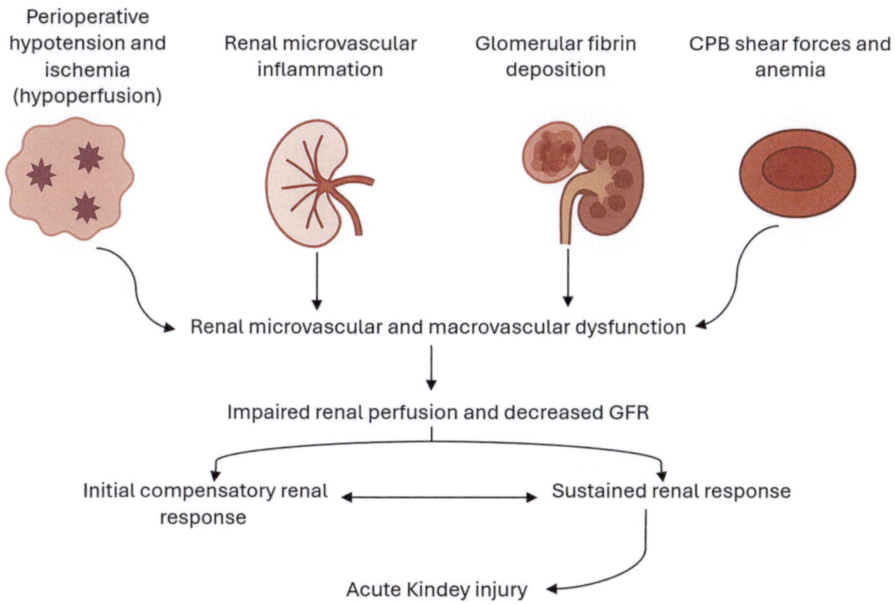

Fig. 1 Factors leading to renal dysfunction during and after cardiopulmonary bypass. Perioperative hypotension, renal microvascular inflammation, glomerular fibrin deposition, and CPB circuit shear forces all act in concert to impair renal perfusion and glomerular filtration rate, ultimately leading to acute kidney injury

2.2 Prevention Measures and Postoperative Care

2.2.1 Preoperative Preventive Strategies

There is no specific pharmacological intervention to prevent CSA-AKI, perioperative pharmacologic prophylaxis strategies remain inconclusive, with corticosteroids, statins, erythropoietin, and sodium bicarbonate showing inconsistent results [49, 50]. Dexmedetomidine may offer nephroprotection, but its use remains debated [51–53]. Atrial natriuretic peptide (ANP) has demonstrated potential benefits in reducing AKI and mortality in cardiac surgery patients [50, 54]. Levosimendan may lower the need for renal replacement therapy (RRT) but requires further validation [50, 55].

To minimize renal injury, nephrotoxic drugs should be avoided during the perioperative period of cardiac surgery. The ERBP Working Group permits a single prophylactic dose of aminoglycosides but advises limiting their use if multiple doses are needed [56].

The preoperative management of ACEis and ARBs remains controversial. While some studies suggest that continuing these medications may reduce AKI risk [57], the 20th ADQI Consensus recommends their perioperative withdrawal [58]. The 2021 ADQI-POQI joint report further suggests stopping ACEis and ARBs at least 24 hours before surgery to prevent perioperative hypotension and postoperative AKI [59]. Although this recommendation primarily targets noncardiac surgeries, it has implications for CSA-AKI.

Both the American ERAS Society [60] and the French Society of Anaesthesia and Intensive Care Medicine (SFAR) [61] recommend initiating prehabilitation at least 4 weeks before cardiac surgery to reduce postoperative complications and hospital stays. A structured prehabilitation program should include patient education, nutritional optimization, exercise training, social support, and anxiety management to enhance functional capacity and improve surgical outcomes.

Current evidence primarily supports the role of preoperative cardiopulmonary and muscle prehabilitation in minimizing pulmonary complications and shortening hospital stays after cardiac surgery [62]. Additionally, studies indicate that prehabilitation exercise therapy before elective abdominal aortic aneurysm repair can lower postoperative serum creatinine levels and reduce the need for hemodialysis or hemofiltration [63]. However, its effectiveness in preventing cardiac surgery-associated acute kidney injury (CSA-AKI) remains uncertain.

2.2.2 Intraoperative Strategies

Optimal Mean Arterial Pressure (MAP)

Maintaining renal perfusion pressure is vital in cardiac surgery. Studies link decreased MAP and increased fluid balance with higher mortality and renal replacement therapy (RRT) needs [64]. Renal autoregulation compensates for MAP changes through the renin-angiotensin-aldosterone system (RAAS) and vasopressin. However, individual variability necessitates personalized hemodynamic monitoring.

Recent data indicate MAP <65 mmHg post-cardiopulmonary bypass (CPB) raises RRT risk [65], though meta-analyses suggest preexisting conditions may contribute more to AKI than intraoperative hypotension [66]. Studies show that raising MAP during CPB does not reduce AKI risk [67]. Current guidelines recommend MAP between 50 and 80 mmHg during CPB [68].

Inotropic and Vasopressor Support

Inotropic agents may be used to improve renal perfusion in cases of low cardiac output, and vasopressors may be used to increase renal perfusion pressure in cases of hypotension. Although vasopressin reduces acute renal failure by 74% in vasoplegic shock compared to norepinephrine [69]. However, ADQI recommends norepinephrine as the primary vasopressor for cardiac surgery [56].

Fluid Management and Goal-Directed Therapy

Fluid management in cardiac surgery is critical, as both fluid overload and hypovolemia contribute to AKI [9]. Studies link a higher positive fluid balance to increased AKI risk and greater RRT requirements [43, 70]. A multicenter study found that while liberal fluid administration did not raise CSA-AKI incidence, it led to higher mortality, more cardiovascular complications, and longer hospital stays [71].

Fluid type also affects AKI risk. Hydroxyethyl starch (HES) increases AKI incidence and is not recommended for high-risk patients [72]. Chloride-rich crystalloids can cause hyperchloremic metabolic acidosis and worsen AKI, while 4% albumin offers no advantage over Ringer acetate [73, 74].

Diuretics are widely used perioperatively but may be harmful. Loop diuretics like furosemide can reduce creatinine clearance, and spironolactone may raise CSA-AKI risk [50]. They are not recommended for AKI prevention but can help manage volume overload [75].

Goal-directed therapy (GDT) optimizes cardiac output using fluids and vasoactive drugs, offering nephroprotective effects and reducing AKI risk post-surgery [76]. It is a *Class I, Level A* recommendation in the *2019 EACTS/EACTA/EBCP* guidelines, supported by strong evidence from RCTs and meta-analyses [77].

Oxygen Delivery in CPB

Adequate oxygen delivery ($DO2 > 260$ mL/min/m^2) during CPB prevents AKI [40]. Goal-directed perfusion (GDP) strategies reduce AKI risk by 50% [78]. Meta-analyses recommend GDP to improve renal outcomes [66].

Transfusion Strategies

Patients undergoing cardiac surgery face a high risk of hemodynamic instability and bleeding, both of which contribute to renal hypoxia. Preoperative anemia is linked to increased AKI and mortality, yet intraoperative packed red blood cell (PRBC) transfusion is also a risk factor for CSA-AKI [79]. Determining the optimal transfusion threshold is crucial.

A restrictive transfusion strategy (maintaining hematocrit ≥24%) showed noninferior 30-day mortality and renal outcomes compared to a liberal strategy (hematocrit ≥30%) [80]. However, large RCTs found no significant difference in AKI incidence between restrictive and liberal transfusion thresholds [81, 82], a finding reinforced by a recent meta-analysis [83]. Current guidelines recommend a PRBC transfusion of Hb <6.0 g/dL [84], with an acceptable hematocrit of 21–24% when DO_2 exceeds 273 mL/min/m^2 [85]. Additionally, red blood cell storage duration does not appear to impact CSA-AKI incidence [86].

Remote Ischemic Preconditioning (RIPC)
RIPC, involving intermittent ischemia-reperfusion cycles, may protect against ischemic injury. Initial studies showed benefit [87], but larger trials did not confirm this [88]. Meta-analyses suggest volatile anesthetics may enhance RIPC efficacy [89], warranting further research.

2.2.3 Postoperative Strategies

The multifactorial nature of CSA-AKI necessitates a structured, guideline-based approach for renal protection. The Kidney Disease: Improving Global Outcomes (KDIGO) guidelines recommend key supportive measures, including discontinuing nephrotoxins, optimizing fluid status and hemodynamics, monitoring serum creatinine (SCr) and urine output, avoiding hyperglycemia, and considering alternatives to radiocontrast procedures [90].

RCTs demonstrated that the KDIGO bundle significantly reduced stage 2 and 3 AKI in high-risk patients [91, 92]. However, compliance was low, with only 65.4% of intervention patients receiving the full bundle, compared to 4.2% in the control group. An observational study across 12 European hospitals further confirmed poor adherence, with just 5.3% of patients receiving all recommended interventions [93].

A meta-analysis found that while the KDIGO bundle did not reduce overall AKI incidence, it significantly lowered severe AKI rates, supporting its use in high-risk patients [66]. The ERAS Society also endorses its implementation, though further trials are needed to improve adherence and confirm its benefits [60].

3 Catheter-Associated Urinary Tract Infections (CAUTI) Post-Cardiac Surgery

Catheter-associated urinary tract infections (CAUTIs) are one of the most common healthcare-associated infections (HAIs), particularly in post-cardiac surgery patients. The presence of an indwelling urinary catheter, coupled with perioperative physiological stress, immunosuppression, and prolonged hospital stays, increases the risk of infection [94]. Despite advancements in surgical techniques and perioperative care, CAUTI remains a significant contributor to morbidity, prolonged hospitalization, and increased healthcare costs [95].

3.1 Risk Factors for CAUTI in Post-Cardiac Surgery Patients

Several factors contribute to the development of CAUTI in patients undergoing cardiac surgery:

1. Prolonged Catheterization
   The duration of urinary catheter use is the most significant risk factor for CAUTI. Studies have shown that the risk of bacteriuria increases by 3–7% per day of catheterization [96]. Post-cardiac surgery patients often require prolonged catheter use due to hemodynamic instability, strict fluid monitoring, and limited mobility.
2. Perioperative Immunosuppression
   Cardiac surgery induces a systemic inflammatory response, leading to transient immunosuppression. The use of cardiopulmonary bypass (CPB) can further impair immune function, predisposing patients to infections, including CAUTI [97, 98].
3. Diabetes Mellitus and Hyperglycemia
   Poor glycemic control is a well-established risk factor for infections in post-surgical patients. Hyperglycemia impairs neutrophil function, delays wound healing, and increases susceptibility to urinary tract infections (UTIs) [98].
4. Renal Dysfunction and Fluid Overload
   Patients with preexisting chronic kidney disease (CKD) or acute kidney injury (AKI) postoperatively have an increased risk of CAUTI. Fluid overload and decreased urine output contribute to urinary stasis, promoting bacterial colonization [99].
5. Prolonged ICU Stay and Mechanical Ventilation
   Critically ill patients in the intensive care unit (ICU) are at heightened risk for CAUTI due to prolonged immobility, increased catheterization duration, and frequent antibiotic exposure, which can alter the urinary microbiome [100].
6. Inappropriate Catheter Care and Handling
   Breaks in aseptic technique during catheter insertion or manipulation can introduce pathogens into the urinary tract, leading to infection. Poor hand hygiene and suboptimal catheter care practices further contribute to CAUTI risk [101].

3.2 Prevention

Preventing CAUTI is critical in post-cardiac surgery patients to reduce morbidity and hospital stay. Key strategies include limiting the overall use of urinary catheters and reducing the duration of catheterization, which are the most effective measures for preventing CAUTI [102–104]. Table 1 outlines measures to reduce the risk of CAUTI among those patients with an ongoing indication for a urinary catheter.

Table 1 Strategies for Prevention of Catheter-Associated Bacteriuria and CAUTI

Before Urinary Catheter Insertion	During Urinary Catheter Insertion	After Urinary Catheter Insertion
Use urinary catheters only when necessary for established indications	Use only trained, dedicated personnel to insert catheters	Remove urinary catheters as soon as no longer indicated
Avoid routine use of urinary catheters for management of incontinence	Perform hand hygiene before and after urinary catheter insertion	Maintain drainage bag and connecting tubing below the level of the bladder
Use portable bladder scanners to assess need for catheterization	Clean urethral meatus with antiseptic solution	Maintain unobstructed urine flow in collecting system
Consider condom catheterization for men without urinary retention	Use aseptic technique and sterile equipment for catheter insertion	Avoid routine catheter irrigation or daily meatal cleansing
Consider intermittent catheterization	Consider use of a preconnected catheter and tubing system	Perform hand hygiene before and after catheter manipulation
	Consider the use of antimicrobial-coated urinary catheters	Properly secure catheters to avoid meatal trauma
		Avoid systemic antibiotic prophylaxis
		Replace catheter and collecting system only for breaks in aseptic technique, disconnection, or leakage

Data derived from Hooton et al. [103], Lo et al. [104], and Fordyce et al. [102]

4 Hematuria in Cardiac Surgery Patients

4.1 Causes and Mechanisms

Hematuria during or after cardiac surgery may arise from preexisting urinary tract conditions, glomerular disease, or anticoagulation-related complications [105]. Anticoagulant-related nephropathy (ARN), commonly linked to warfarin and non-vitamin K antagonist oral anticoagulants (NOACs) like dabigatran and rivaroxaban, can cause gross hematuria and AKI, particularly when the international normalized ratio (INR) >3 [106, 107]. ARN results from thrombin depletion and endothelial dysfunction, leading to glomerular hemorrhage and renal tubular obstruction [108].

Drug-induced acute interstitial nephritis (DAIN) is another cause, triggered by commonly used perioperative medications, including β-lactam antibiotics, vancomycin, diuretics, and proton pump inhibitors. DAIN manifests with microscopic hematuria in two-thirds of cases and gross hematuria in 5% of patients. Up to 70% of affected individuals experience incomplete renal recovery, with some requiring dialysis [109–111].

Hematuria may also result from catheter-induced urethral trauma or suprapubic cystostomy, particularly in anticoagulated patients [110, 112, 113]. The European Association of Cardiothoracic Surgery recommends discontinuing warfarin 5 days before elective surgery and stopping NOACs at least 48 hours prior, depending on renal function [113].

Patients on ventricular assist devices (VADs) or extracorporeal membrane oxygenation (ECMO) may develop acquired von Willebrand syndrome (VWS), leading to hematuria due to mucosal bleeding. This is attributed to the loss of high-molecular-weight von Willebrand factor (VWF) multimers, impairing platelet adhesion [114].

4.2 Management and Treatment

Treatment depends on the underlying cause. Urology referral is warranted for structural urinary tract pathology, while immunosuppressive therapy may be considered for immune-mediated glomerular diseases [115]. Corticosteroids, iron chelators, diuretics, and antioxidants like N-acetylcysteine have shown potential in mitigating renal damage in ARN [115–117].

For ARN, switching from warfarin to an NOAC or reducing NOAC dosage is advised. DAIN requires prompt identification and discontinuation of the offending drug, with kidney biopsy indicated if renal function does not improve within 5 days. Early steroid use may reduce inflammation and long-term renal impairment [109, 111, 116, 118]. In cases of acquired VWS, management includes desmopressin, VWF-containing concentrates, plasmapheresis, or recombinant factor VIIa to control severe bleeding [119].

References

1. Block CA, Schoolwerth AC. The epidemiology and outcome of acute renal failure and the impact on chronic kidney disease. Semin Dial. 2006;19(6):450–4. https://doi.org/10.1111/j.1525-139X.2006.00206.x.
2. Boyer N, Eldridge J, Prowle JR, Forni LG. Postoperative acute kidney injury. Clin J Am Soc Nephrol. 2022;17(10):1535–45. https://doi.org/10.2215/CJN.16541221.
3. Hobson CE, Yavas S, Segal MS, Schold JD, Tribble CG, Layon AJ, Bihorac A. Acute kidney injury is associated with increased long-term mortality after cardiothoracic surgery. Circulation. 2009;119(18):2444–53. https://doi.org/10.1161/CIRCULATIONAHA.108.800011.
4. Kellum JA, Hoste EA. Acute kidney injury: epidemiology and assessment. Scand J Clin Lab Invest Suppl. 2008;241:6–11. https://doi.org/10.1080/00365510802144813.
5. Kellum JA, Prowle JR. Paradigms of acute kidney injury in the intensive care setting. Nat Rev Nephrol. 2018;14(4):217–30. https://doi.org/10.1038/nrneph.2017.184.
6. Neild GH. Multi-organ renal failure in the elderly. Int Urol Nephrol. 2001;32(4):559–65. https://doi.org/10.1023/a:1014474305423.
7. Peerapornratana S, Manrique-Caballero CL, Gomez H, Kellum JA. Acute kidney injury from sepsis: current concepts, epidemiology, pathophysiology, prevention and treatment. Kidney Int. 2019;96(5):1083–99. https://doi.org/10.1016/j.kint.2019.05.026.

8. Waikar SS, Liu KD, Chertow GM. Diagnosis, epidemiology and outcomes of acute kidney injury. Clin J Am Soc Nephrol. 2008;3(3):844–61. https://doi.org/10.2215/CJN.05191107.
9. Wang Y, Bellomo R. Cardiac surgery-associated acute kidney injury: risk factors, pathophysiology and treatment. Nat Rev Nephrol. 2017;13(11):697–711. https://doi.org/10.1038/nrneph.2017.119.
10. Axtell AL, Fiedler AG, Melnitchouk S, D'Alessandro DA, Villavicencio MA, Jassar AS, Sundt TM 3rd. Correlation of cardiopulmonary bypass duration with acute renal failure after cardiac surgery. J Thorac Cardiovasc Surg. 2020;159(1):170–178 e172. https://doi.org/10.1016/j.jtcvs.2019.01.072.
11. Grams ME, Sang Y, Coresh J, Ballew S, Matsushita K, Molnar MZ, et al. Acute kidney injury after major surgery: a retrospective analysis of veterans health administration data. Am J Kidney Dis. 2016;67(6):872–80. https://doi.org/10.1053/j.ajkd.2015.07.022.
12. Ishani A, Nelson D, Clothier B, Schult T, Nugent S, Greer N, et al. The magnitude of acute serum creatinine increase after cardiac surgery and the risk of chronic kidney disease, progression of kidney disease, and death. Arch Intern Med. 2011;171(3):226–33. https://doi.org/10.1001/archinternmed.2010.514.
13. Corredor C, Thomson R, Al-Subaie N. Long-term consequences of acute kidney injury after cardiac surgery: a systematic review and meta-analysis. J Cardiothorac Vasc Anesth. 2016;30(1):69–75. https://doi.org/10.1053/j.jvca.2015.07.013.
14. Hu J, Chen R, Liu S, Yu X, Zou J, Ding X. Global incidence and outcomes of adult patients with acute kidney injury after cardiac surgery: a systematic review and meta-analysis. J Cardiothorac Vasc Anesth. 2016;30(1):82–9. https://doi.org/10.1053/j.jvca.2015.06.017.
15. Fuhrman DY, Kellum JA. Epidemiology and pathophysiology of cardiac surgery-associated acute kidney injury. Curr Opin Anaesthesiol. 2017;30(1):60–5. https://doi.org/10.1097/ACO.0000000000000412.
16. Rosner MH, Okusa MD. Acute kidney injury associated with cardiac surgery. Clin J Am Soc Nephrol. 2006;1(1):19–32. https://doi.org/10.2215/CJN.00240605.
17. Goldfarb DW. Points to remember: frequently encountered urologic problems after cardiovascular surgery. Methodist Debakey Cardiovasc J. 2014;10(2):131–2. https://doi.org/10.14797/mdcj-10-2-131.
18. Bellini MI, Charalampidis S, Herbert PE, Bonatsos V, Crane J, Muthusamy A, et al. Cold pulsatile machine perfusion versus static cold storage in kidney transplantation: a single centre experience. Biomed Res Int. 2019;2019:7435248. https://doi.org/10.1155/2019/7435248.
19. Sgouralis I, Evans RG, Layton AT. Renal medullary and urinary oxygen tension during cardiopulmonary bypass in the rat. Math Med Biol. 2017;34(3):313–33. https://doi.org/10.1093/imammb/dqw010.
20. Sreeram GM, Grocott HP, White WD, Newman MF, Stafford-Smith M. Transcranial Doppler emboli count predicts rise in creatinine after coronary artery bypass graft surgery. J Cardiothorac Vasc Anesth. 2004;18(5):548–51. https://doi.org/10.1053/j.jvca.2004.07.010.
21. Vermeulen Windsant IC, de Wit NC, Sertorio JT, van Bijnen AA, Ganushchak YM, Heijmans JH, et al. Hemolysis during cardiac surgery is associated with increased intravascular nitric oxide consumption and perioperative kidney and intestinal tissue damage. Front Physiol. 2014;5:340. https://doi.org/10.3389/fphys.2014.00340.
22. Sutton TA, Fisher CJ, Molitoris BA. Microvascular endothelial injury and dysfunction during ischemic acute renal failure. Kidney Int. 2002;62(5):1539–49. https://doi.org/10.1046/j.1523-1755.2002.00631.x.
23. Ronco C, Bellomo R, Kellum JA. Acute kidney injury. Lancet. 2019;394(10212):1949–64. https://doi.org/10.1016/S0140-6736(19)32563-2.
24. Che M, Wang X, Liu S, Xie B, Xue S, Yan Y, et al. A clinical score to predict severe acute kidney injury in Chinese patients after cardiac surgery. Nephron. 2019;142(4):291–300. https://doi.org/10.1159/000499345.
25. Chen L, Hong L, Ma A, Chen Y, Xiao Y, Jiang F, et al. Intraoperative venous congestion rather than hypotension is associated with acute adverse kidney events after cardiac surgery:

a retrospective cohort study. Br J Anaesth. 2022;128(5):785–95. https://doi.org/10.1016/j.bja.2022.01.032.

26. Mukaida H, Matsushita S, Yamamoto T, Minami Y, Sato G, Asai T, Amano A. Oxygen delivery-guided perfusion for the prevention of acute kidney injury: a randomized controlled trial. J Thorac Cardiovasc Surg. 2023;165(2):750–760 e755. https://doi.org/10.1016/j.jtcvs.2021.03.032.
27. Su L, Zhang J, Gomez H, Kellum JA, Peng Z. Mitochondria ROS and mitophagy in acute kidney injury. Autophagy. 2023;19(2):401–14. https://doi.org/10.1080/15548627.2022.2084862.
28. Asimakopoulos G, Taylor KM. Effects of cardiopulmonary bypass on leukocyte and endothelial adhesion molecules. Ann Thorac Surg. 1998;66(6):2135–44. https://doi.org/10.1016/s0003-4975(98)00727-9.
29. Westaby S. Complement and the damaging effects of cardiopulmonary bypass. Thorax. 1983;38(5):321–5. https://doi.org/10.1136/thx.38.5.321.
30. Presta P, Bolignano D, Coppolino G, Serraino F, Mastroroberto P, Andreucci M, Fuiano G. Antecedent ACE-inhibition, inflammatory response, and cardiac surgery associated acute kidney injury. Rev Cardiovasc Med. 2021;22(1):207–13. https://doi.org/10.31083/j.rcm.2021.01.288.
31. Wu MY, Yiang GT, Liao WT, Tsai AP, Cheng YL, Cheng PW, et al. Current mechanistic concepts in ischemia and reperfusion injury. Cell Physiol Biochem. 2018;46(4):1650–67. https://doi.org/10.1159/000489241.
32. Bonventre JV, Yang L. Cellular pathophysiology of ischemic acute kidney injury. J Clin Invest. 2011;121(11):4210–21. https://doi.org/10.1172/JCI45161.
33. Hatami S, Hefler J, Freed DH. Inflammation and oxidative stress in the context of extracorporeal cardiac and pulmonary support. Front Immunol. 2022;13:831930. https://doi.org/10.3389/fimmu.2022.831930.
34. Moat NE, Evans TE, Quinlan GJ, Gutteridge JM. Chelatable iron and copper can be released from extracorporeally circulated blood during cardiopulmonary bypass. FEBS Lett. 1993;328(1–2):103–6. https://doi.org/10.1016/0014-5793(93)80974-y.
35. Haase M, Bellomo R, Haase-Fielitz A. Novel biomarkers, oxidative stress, and the role of labile iron toxicity in cardiopulmonary bypass-associated acute kidney injury. J Am Coll Cardiol. 2010;55(19):2024–33. https://doi.org/10.1016/j.jacc.2009.12.046.
36. Horl WH. Nonsteroidal anti-inflammatory drugs and the kidney. Pharmaceuticals (Basel). 2010;3(7):2291–321. https://doi.org/10.3390/ph3072291.
37. O'Neal JB, Shaw AD, Billings FT. Acute kidney injury following cardiac surgery: current understanding and future directions. Crit Care. 2016;20(1):187. https://doi.org/10.1186/s13054-016-1352-z.
38. Nielsen DV, Hjortdal V, Larsson H, Johnsen SP, Jakobsen CJ. Perioperative aminoglycoside treatment is associated with a higher incidence of postoperative dialysis in adult cardiac surgery patients. J Thorac Cardiovasc Surg. 2011;142(3):656–61. https://doi.org/10.1016/j.jtcvs.2011.03.019.
39. Lombardi R, Ferreiro A, Servetto C. Renal function after cardiac surgery: adverse effect of furosemide. Ren Fail. 2003;25(5):775–86. https://doi.org/10.1081/jdi-120024293.
40. Ranucci M, Ballotta A, Kunkl A, De Benedetti D, Kandil H, Conti D, et al. Influence of the timing of cardiac catheterization and the amount of contrast media on acute renal failure after cardiac surgery. Am J Cardiol. 2008;101(8):1112–8. https://doi.org/10.1016/j.amjcard.2007.12.011.
41. Schrier RW, Abraham WT. Hormones and hemodynamics in heart failure. N Engl J Med. 1999;341(8):577–85. https://doi.org/10.1056/NEJM199908193410806.
42. Yu Y, Li C, Zhu S, Jin L, Hu Y, Ling X, et al. Diagnosis, pathophysiology and preventive strategies for cardiac surgery-associated acute kidney injury: a narrative review. Eur J Med Res. 2023;28(1):45. https://doi.org/10.1186/s40001-023-00990-2.

43. Haase M, Haase-Fielitz A, Bagshaw SM, Ronco C, Bellomo R. Cardiopulmonary bypass-associated acute kidney injury: a pigment nephropathy? Contrib Nephrol. 2007;156:340–53. https://doi.org/10.1159/000102125.
44. Scindia Y, Dey P, Thirunagari A, Liping H, Rosin DL, Floris M, et al. Hepcidin mitigates renal ischemia-reperfusion injury by modulating systemic iron homeostasis. J Am Soc Nephrol. 2015;26(11):2800–14. https://doi.org/10.1681/ASN.2014101037.
45. Sharma S, Leaf DE. Iron chelation as a potential therapeutic strategy for AKI prevention. J Am Soc Nephrol. 2019;30(11):2060–71. https://doi.org/10.1681/ASN.2019060595.
46. Boehm J, Eichhorn S, Kornek M, Hauner K, Prinzing A, Grammer J, et al. Apolipoprotein E genotype, TNF-alpha 308G/A and risk for cardiac surgery associated-acute kidney injury in Caucasians. Ren Fail. 2014;36(2):237–43. https://doi.org/10.3109/0886022X.2013.835267.
47. Kornek M, Deutsch MA, Eichhorn S, Lahm H, Wagenpfeil S, Krane M, et al. COMT-Val158Met-polymorphism is not a risk factor for acute kidney injury after cardiac surgery. Dis Markers. 2013;35(2):129–34. https://doi.org/10.1155/2013/279046.
48. Ortega-Loubon C, Martinez-Paz P, Garcia-Moran E, Tamayo-Velasco A, Lopez-Hernandez FJ, Jorge-Monjas P, Tamayo E. Genetic susceptibility to acute kidney injury. J Clin Med. 2021;10(14) https://doi.org/10.3390/jcm10143039.
49. Ostermann M, Kunst G, Baker E, Weerapolchai K, Lumlertgul N. Cardiac surgery associated AKI prevention strategies and medical treatment for CSA-AKI. J Clin Med. 2021;10(22) https://doi.org/10.3390/jcm10225285.
50. Pathak S, Olivieri G, Mohamed W, Abbasciano R, Roman M, Tomassini S, et al. Pharmacological interventions for the prevention of renal injury in surgical patients: a systematic literature review and meta-analysis. Br J Anaesth. 2021;126(1):131–8. https://doi.org/10.1016/j.bja.2020.06.064.
51. Gu J, Sun P, Zhao H, Watts HR, Sanders RD, Terrando N, et al. Dexmedetomidine provides renoprotection against ischemia-reperfusion injury in mice. Crit Care. 2011;15(3):R153. https://doi.org/10.1186/cc10283.
52. Peng K, Li D, Applegate RL 2nd, Lubarsky DA, Ji FH, Liu H. Effect of dexmedetomidine on cardiac surgery-associated acute kidney injury: a meta-analysis with trial sequential analysis of randomized controlled trials. J Cardiothorac Vasc Anesth. 2020;34(3):603–13. https://doi.org/10.1053/j.jvca.2019.09.011.
53. Turan A, Duncan A, Leung S, Karimi N, Fang J, Mao G, et al. Dexmedetomidine for reduction of atrial fibrillation and delirium after cardiac surgery (DECADE): a randomised placebo-controlled trial. Lancet. 2020;396(10245):177–85. https://doi.org/10.1016/S0140-6736(20)30631-0.
54. Nigwekar SU, Navaneethan SD, Parikh CR, Hix JK. Atrial natriuretic peptide for preventing and treating acute kidney injury. Cochrane Database Syst Rev. 2009;(4):CD006028. https://doi.org/10.1002/14651858.CD006028.pub2.
55. Landoni G, Lomivorotov VV, Alvaro G, Lobreglio R, Pisano A, Guarracino F, et al. Levosimendan for hemodynamic support after cardiac surgery. N Engl J Med. 2017;376(21):2021–31. https://doi.org/10.1056/NEJMoa1616325.
56. Ad-hoc working group of E, Fliser D, Laville M, Covic A, Fouque D, Vanholder R, et al. A European Renal Best Practice (ERBP) position statement on the Kidney Disease Improving Global Outcomes (KDIGO) clinical practice guidelines on acute kidney injury: part 1: definitions, conservative management and contrast-induced nephropathy. Nephrol Dial Transplant. 2012;27(12):4263–72. https://doi.org/10.1093/ndt/gfs375.
57. Coca SG, Garg AX, Swaminathan M, Garwood S, Hong K, Thiessen-Philbrook H, et al. Preoperative angiotensin-converting enzyme inhibitors and angiotensin receptor blocker use and acute kidney injury in patients undergoing cardiac surgery. Nephrol Dial Transplant. 2013;28(11):2787–99. https://doi.org/10.1093/ndt/gft405.
58. Nadim MK, Forni LG, Bihorac A, Hobson C, Koyner JL, Shaw A, et al. Cardiac and vascular surgery-associated acute kidney injury: the 20th International Consensus Conference of the ADQI (acute disease quality initiative) group. J Am Heart Assoc. 2018;7(11) https://doi.org/10.1161/JAHA.118.008834.

59. Prowle JR, Forni LG, Bell M, Chew MS, Edwards M, Grams ME, et al. Postoperative acute kidney injury in adult non-cardiac surgery: joint consensus report of the acute disease quality initiative and perioperative quality initiative. Nat Rev Nephrol. 2021;17(9):605–18. https://doi.org/10.1038/s41581-021-00418-2.
60. Engelman DT, Ben Ali W, Williams JB, Perrault LP, Reddy VS, Arora RC, et al. Guidelines for perioperative care in cardiac surgery: enhanced recovery after surgery society recommendations. JAMA Surg. 2019;154(8):755–66. https://doi.org/10.1001/jamasurg.2019.1153.
61. Mertes PM, Kindo M, Amour J, Baufreton C, Camilleri L, Caus T, et al. Guidelines on enhanced recovery after cardiac surgery under cardiopulmonary bypass or off-pump. Anaesth Crit Care Pain Med. 2022;41(3):101059. https://doi.org/10.1016/j.accpm.2022.101059.
62. Nardi P, Pisano C, Altieri C, Buioni D, Pedicelli C, Saulle S, et al. The benefit of a preoperative respiratory protocol and musculoskeletal exercise in patients undergoing cardiac surgery. Kardiochir Torakochirurgia Pol. 2020;17(2):94–100. https://doi.org/10.5114/kitp.2020.97267.
63. Fenton C, Tan AR, Abaraogu UO, McCaslin JE. Prehabilitation exercise therapy before elective abdominal aortic aneurysm repair. Cochrane Database Syst Rev. 2021;7(7):CD013662. https://doi.org/10.1002/14651858.CD013662.pub2.
64. Haase-Fielitz A, Haase M, Bellomo R, Calzavacca P, Spura A, Baraki H, et al. Perioperative hemodynamic instability and fluid overload are associated with increasing acute kidney injury severity and worse outcome after cardiac surgery. Blood Purif. 2017;43(4):298–308. https://doi.org/10.1159/000455061.
65. Ngu JMC, Jabagi H, Chung AM, Boodhwani M, Ruel M, Bourke M, Sun LY. Defining an intraoperative hypotension threshold in association with De Novo Renal replacement therapy after cardiac surgery. Anesthesiology. 2020;132(6):1447–57. https://doi.org/10.1097/ALN.0000000000003254.
66. Peng K, McIlroy DR, Bollen BA, Billings FTT, Zarbock A, Popescu WM, et al. Society of cardiovascular anesthesiologists clinical practice update for management of acute kidney injury associated with cardiac surgery. Anesth Analg. 2022;135(4):744–56. https://doi.org/10.1213/ANE.0000000000006068.
67. Kofford B, Drago C, Nejat AH, Elshewy M. A novel approach for converting a mandibular complete denture to a fixed interim, screw-retained implant prostheses: a case report. J Prosthodont. 2021;30(1):13–8. https://doi.org/10.1111/jopr.13285.
68. Vedel AG, Holmgaard F, Rasmussen LS, Langkilde A, Paulson OB, Lange T, et al. High-target versus low-target blood pressure management during cardiopulmonary bypass to prevent cerebral injury in cardiac surgery patients: a randomized controlled trial. Circulation. 2018;137(17):1770–80. https://doi.org/10.1161/CIRCULATIONAHA.117.030308.
69. Hajjar LA, Vincent JL, Barbosa Gomes Galas FR, Rhodes A, Landoni G, Osawa EA, et al. Vasopressin versus norepinephrine in patients with Vasoplegic shock after cardiac surgery: the VANCS randomized controlled trial. Anesthesiology. 2017;126(1):85–93. https://doi.org/10.1097/ALN.0000000000001434.
70. Shen Y, Zhang W, Cheng X, Ying M. Association between postoperative fluid balance and acute kidney injury in patients after cardiac surgery: a retrospective cohort study. J Crit Care. 2018;44:273–7. https://doi.org/10.1016/j.jcrc.2017.11.041.
71. Palomba H, Treml RE, Caldonazo T, Katayama HT, Gomes BC, Malbouisson LMS, Silva Junior JM. Intraoperative fluid balance and cardiac surgery-associated acute kidney injury: a multicenter prospective study. Braz J Anesthesiol. 2022;72(6):688–94. https://doi.org/10.1016/j.bjane.2022.07.006.
72. Glassford NJ, French CJ, Bailey M, Mårtensson J, Eastwood GM, Bellomo R. Changes in intravenous fluid use patterns in Australia and New Zealand: evidence of research translating into practice. Crit Care Resusc. 2016;18(2):78–88. https://doi.org/10.1016/s1441-2772(23)01009-8.
73. Bhaskaran K, Arumugam G, Vinay Kumar PV. A prospective, randomized, comparison study on effect of perioperative use of chloride liberal intravenous fluids versus chloride restricted intravenous fluids on postoperative acute kidney injury in patients undergoing off-pump

coronary artery bypass grafting surgeries. Ann Card Anaesth. 2018;21(4):413–8. https://doi.org/10.4103/aca.ACA_230_17.
74. Pesonen E, Vlasov H, Suojaranta R, Hiippala S, Schramko A, Wilkman E, et al. Effect of 4% albumin solution vs ringer acetate on major adverse events in patients undergoing cardiac surgery with cardiopulmonary bypass: a randomized clinical trial. JAMA. 2022;328(3):251–8. https://doi.org/10.1001/jama.2022.10461.
75. Khwaja A. KDIGO clinical practice guidelines for acute kidney injury. Nephron Clin Pract. 2012;120(4):c179–84. https://doi.org/10.1159/000339789.
76. Magruder JT, Crawford TC, Harness HL, Grimm JC, Suarez-Pierre A, Wierschke C, et al. A pilot goal-directed perfusion initiative is associated with less acute kidney injury after cardiac surgery. J Thorac Cardiovasc Surg. 2017;153(1):118–125 e111. https://doi.org/10.1016/j.jtcvs.2016.09.016.
77. Authors/Task Force, M, Kunst G, Milojevic M, Boer C, De Somer F, Gudbjartsson T, et al. 2019 EACTS/EACTA/EBCP guidelines on cardiopulmonary bypass in adult cardiac surgery. Br J Anaesth. 2019;123(6):713–57. https://doi.org/10.1016/j.bja.2019.09.012.
78. Ranucci M, Johnson I, Willcox T, Baker RA, Boer C, Baumann A, et al. Goal-directed perfusion to reduce acute kidney injury: a randomized trial. J Thorac Cardiovasc Surg. 2018;156(5):1918–1927 e1912. https://doi.org/10.1016/j.jtcvs.2018.04.045.
79. Oprea AD, Del Rio JM, Cooter M, Green CL, Karhausen JA, Nailer P, et al. Pre- and post-operative anemia, acute kidney injury, and mortality after coronary artery bypass grafting surgery: a retrospective observational study. Can J Anaesth. 2018;65(1):46–59. https://doi.org/10.1007/s12630-017-0991-0.
80. Hajjar LA, Vincent JL, Galas FR, Nakamura RE, Silva CM, Santos MH, et al. Transfusion requirements after cardiac surgery: the TRACS randomized controlled trial. JAMA. 2010;304(14):1559–67. https://doi.org/10.1001/jama.2010.1446.
81. Garg AX, Badner N, Bagshaw SM, Cuerden MS, Fergusson DA, Gregory AJ, et al. Safety of a restrictive versus liberal approach to red blood cell transfusion on the outcome of AKI in patients undergoing cardiac surgery: a randomized clinical trial. J Am Soc Nephrol. 2019;30(7):1294–304. https://doi.org/10.1681/ASN.2019010004.
82. Mazer CD, Whitlock RP, Fergusson DA, Hall J, Belley-Cote E, Connolly K, et al. Restrictive or liberal red-cell transfusion for cardiac surgery. N Engl J Med. 2017;377(22):2133–44. https://doi.org/10.1056/NEJMoa1711818.
83. Chen QH, Wang HL, Liu L, Shao J, Yu J, Zheng RQ. Effects of restrictive red blood cell transfusion on the prognoses of adult patients undergoing cardiac surgery: a meta-analysis of randomized controlled trials. Crit Care. 2018;22(1):142. https://doi.org/10.1186/s13054-018-2062-5.
84. Society of Thoracic Surgeons Blood Conservation Guideline Task, F, Ferraris VA, Brown JR, Despotis GJ, Hammon JW, Reece TB, et al. 2011 update to the Society of Thoracic Surgeons and the Society of Cardiovascular Anesthesiologists blood conservation clinical practice guidelines. Ann Thorac Surg. 2011;91(3):944–82. https://doi.org/10.1016/j.athoracsur.2010.11.078.
85. Pagano D, Milojevic M, Meesters MI, Benedetto U, Bolliger D, von Heymann C, et al. 2017 EACTS/EACTA guidelines on patient blood management for adult cardiac surgery. Eur J Cardiothorac Surg. 2018;53(1):79–111. https://doi.org/10.1093/ejcts/ezx325.
86. Steiner ME, Ness PM, Assmann SF, Triulzi DJ, Sloan SR, Delaney M, et al. Effects of red-cell storage duration on patients undergoing cardiac surgery. N Engl J Med. 2015;372(15):1419–29. https://doi.org/10.1056/NEJMoa1414219.
87. Zarbock A, Schmidt C, Van Aken H, Wempe C, Martens S, Zahn PK, et al. Effect of remote ischemic preconditioning on kidney injury among high-risk patients undergoing cardiac surgery: a randomized clinical trial. JAMA. 2015;313(21):2133–41. https://doi.org/10.1001/jama.2015.4189.
88. Hausenloy DJ, Candilio L, Evans R, Ariti C, Jenkins DP, Kolvekar S, et al. Remote ischemic preconditioning and outcomes of cardiac surgery. N Engl J Med. 2015;373(15):1408–17. https://doi.org/10.1056/NEJMoa1413534.

89. Xie J, Zhang X, Xu J, Zhang Z, Klingensmith NJ, Liu S, et al. Effect of remote ischemic preconditioning on outcomes in adult cardiac surgery: a systematic review and meta-analysis of randomized controlled studies. Anesth Analg. 2018;127(1):30–8. https://doi.org/10.1213/ane.0000000000002674.
90. Kellum JA, Lameire N, Group KAGW. Diagnosis, evaluation, and management of acute kidney injury: a KDIGO summary (Part 1). Crit Care. 2013;17(1):204. https://doi.org/10.1186/cc11454.
91. Meersch M, Schmidt C, Hoffmeier A, Van Aken H, Wempe C, Gerss J, Zarbock A. Prevention of cardiac surgery-associated AKI by implementing the KDIGO guidelines in high risk patients identified by biomarkers: the PrevAKI randomized controlled trial. Intensive Care Med. 2017;43(11):1551–61. https://doi.org/10.1007/s00134-016-4670-3.
92. Zarbock A, Kullmar M, Ostermann M, Lucchese G, Baig K, Cennamo A, et al. Prevention of cardiac surgery-associated acute kidney injury by implementing the KDIGO guidelines in high-risk patients identified by biomarkers: the PrevAKI-multicenter randomized controlled trial. Anesth Analg. 2021;133(2):292–302. https://doi.org/10.1213/ANE.0000000000005458.
93. Kullmar M, Weiss R, Ostermann M, Campos S, Grau Novellas N, Thomson G, et al. A multinational observational study exploring adherence with the kidney disease: improving global outcomes recommendations for prevention of acute kidney injury after cardiac surgery. Anesth Analg. 2020;130(4):910–6. https://doi.org/10.1213/ANE.0000000000004642.
94. Krein SL, Saint S, Trautner BW, Kuhn L, Colozzi J, Ratz D, et al. Patient-reported complications related to peripherally inserted central catheters: a multicentre prospective cohort study. BMJ Qual Saf. 2019;28(7):574–81. https://doi.org/10.1136/bmjqs-2018-008726.
95. Werneburg GT. Catheter-associated urinary tract infections: current challenges and future prospects. Res Rep Urol. 2022;14:109–33. https://doi.org/10.2147/RRU.S273663.
96. Klevens RM, Edwards JR, Richards CL Jr, Horan TC, Gaynes RP, Pollock DA, Cardo DM. Estimating health care-associated infections and deaths in U.S. hospitals, 2002. Public Health Rep. 2007;122(2):160–6. https://doi.org/10.1177/003335490712200205.
97. Gaudriot B, Uhel F, Gregoire M, Gacouin A, Biedermann S, Roisne A, et al. Immune dysfunction after cardiac surgery with cardiopulmonary bypass: beneficial effects of maintaining mechanical ventilation. Shock. 2015;44(3):228–33. https://doi.org/10.1097/SHK.0000000000000416.
98. Gillen JR, Isbell JM, Michaels AD, Lau CL, Sawyer RG. Risk factors for urinary tract infections in cardiac surgical patients. Surg Infect. 2015;16(5):504–8. https://doi.org/10.1089/sur.2013.115.
99. Funfstuck R, Ott U, Naber KG. The interaction of urinary tract infection and renal insufficiency. Int J Antimicrob Agents. 2006;28(Suppl 1):S72–7. https://doi.org/10.1016/j.ijantimicag.2006.05.004.
100. Rabi R, Enaya A, Jomaa DM, Dweekat MZ, Raddad S, Saqfalhait ZT, Abu-Gaber D. Catheter-associated urinary tract infections in critical care: understanding incidence, risk factors, and pathogenic causes in Palestine. PLoS One. 2024;19(8):e0309755. https://doi.org/10.1371/journal.pone.0309755.
101. Saint S, Greene MT, Krein SL, Rogers MA, Ratz D, Fowler KE, et al. A program to prevent catheter-associated urinary tract infection in acute care. N Engl J Med. 2016;374(22):2111–9. https://doi.org/10.1056/NEJMoa1504906.
102. Fordyce CB, Katz JN, Alviar CL, Arslanian-Engoren C, Bohula EA, Geller BJ, et al. Prevention of complications in the cardiac intensive care unit: a scientific statement from the American Heart Association. Circulation. 2020;142(22):e379–406. https://doi.org/10.1161/CIR.0000000000000909.
103. Hooton TM, Bradley SF, Cardenas DD, Colgan R, Geerlings SE, Rice JC, et al. Diagnosis, prevention, and treatment of catheter-associated urinary tract infection in adults: 2009 International Clinical Practice Guidelines from the Infectious Diseases Society of America. Clin Infect Dis. 2010;50(5):625–63. https://doi.org/10.1086/650482.

104. Lo E, Nicolle LE, Coffin SE, Gould C, Maragakis LL, Meddings J, et al. Strategies to prevent catheter-associated urinary tract infections in acute care hospitals: 2014 update. Infect Control Hosp Epidemiol. 2014;35(5):464–79. https://doi.org/10.1086/675718.
105. Veerreddy P. Hemoglobinuria misidentified as hematuria: review of discolored urine and paroxysmal nocturnal hemoglobinuria. Clin Med Insights Blood Disord. 2013;6:7–17. https://doi.org/10.4137/CMBD.S11517.
106. Brodsky S, Eikelboom J, Hebert LA. Anticoagulant-related nephropathy. J Am Soc Nephrol. 2018;29(12):2787–93. https://doi.org/10.1681/ASN.2018070741.
107. Brodsky SV, Satoskar A, Chen J, Nadasdy G, Eagen JW, Hamirani M, et al. Acute kidney injury during warfarin therapy associated with obstructive tubular red blood cell casts: a report of 9 cases. Am J Kidney Dis. 2009;54(6):1121–6. https://doi.org/10.1053/j.ajkd.2009.04.024.
108. Ware K, Brodsky P, Satoskar AA, Nadasdy T, Nadasdy G, Wu H, et al. Warfarin-related nephropathy modeled by nephron reduction and excessive anticoagulation. J Am Soc Nephrol. 2011;22(10):1856–62. https://doi.org/10.1681/ASN.2010101110.
109. Gonzalez E, Gutierrez E, Galeano C, Chevia C, de Sequera P, Bernis C, et al. Early steroid treatment improves the recovery of renal function in patients with drug-induced acute interstitial nephritis. Kidney Int. 2008;73(8):940–6. https://doi.org/10.1038/sj.ki.5002776.
110. Koh LY, Hwang NC. Red-colored urine in the cardiac surgical patient-diagnosis, causes, and management. J Cardiothorac Vasc Anesth. 2021;35(12):3774–88. https://doi.org/10.1053/j.jvca.2020.10.014.
111. Praga M, Gonzalez E. Acute interstitial nephritis. Kidney Int. 2010;77(11):956–61. https://doi.org/10.1038/ki.2010.89.
112. Konttinen M, Alfthan O, Heikkinen L, Jarvinen A, Ruutu M. Suprapubic cystostomy catheterization in open-heart surgery. Scand J Thorac Cardiovasc Surg. 1984;18(2):167–8. https://doi.org/10.3109/14017438409102400.
113. Sousa-Uva M, Head SJ, Milojevic M, Collet JP, Landoni G, Castella M, et al. 2017 EACTS guidelines on perioperative medication in adult cardiac surgery. Eur J Cardiothorac Surg. 2018;53(1):5–33. https://doi.org/10.1093/ejcts/ezx314.
114. Rauch A, Susen S, Zieger B. Acquired von Willebrand syndrome in patients with ventricular assist device. Front Med (Lausanne). 2019;6:7. https://doi.org/10.3389/fmed.2019.00007.
115. Moreno JA, Sevillano A, Gutierrez E, Guerrero-Hue M, Vazquez-Carballo C, Yuste C, et al. Glomerular hematuria: cause or consequence of renal inflammation? Int J Mol Sci. 2019;20(9) https://doi.org/10.3390/ijms20092205.
116. Lin Y, Jia J, Guo Y, He D, Zhang Y, Wang F, et al. Corticosteroid for IgA nephropathy: are they really therapeutic? Am J Nephrol. 2018;47(6):385–94. https://doi.org/10.1159/000489580.
117. Ware K, Qamri Z, Ozcan A, Satoskar AA, Nadasdy G, Rovin BH, et al. N-acetylcysteine ameliorates acute kidney injury but not glomerular hemorrhage in an animal model of warfarin-related nephropathy. Am J Physiol Renal Physiol. 2013;304(12):F1421–7. https://doi.org/10.1152/ajprenal.00689.2012.
118. Clarkson MR, Giblin L, O'Connell FP, O'Kelly P, Walshe JJ, Conlon P, et al. Acute interstitial nephritis: clinical features and response to corticosteroid therapy. Nephrol Dial Transplant. 2004;19(11):2778–83. https://doi.org/10.1093/ndt/gfh485.
119. Kalbhenn J, Schmidt R, Nakamura L, Schelling J, Rosenfelder S, Zieger B. Early diagnosis of acquired von Willebrand Syndrome (AVWS) is elementary for clinical practice in patients treated with ECMO therapy. J Atheroscler Thromb. 2015;22(3):265–71. https://doi.org/10.5551/jat.27268.

Postoperative Respiratory Care, Including Pleural Space Complications

Ma'in Al Shawabkeh, Mohamed Elmestekawy, and Anas N. Shallik

1 Introduction

Cardiac surgery, though lifesaving, carries the risk of various pulmonary complications that can profoundly influence patient outcomes. Among the most common are atelectasis, pleural effusion, acute respiratory distress syndrome (ARDS), pneumonia, phrenic nerve injury, diaphragmatic dysfunction, and pneumothorax—each arising from distinct intraoperative and postoperative factors—resulting in prolonged hospital stays, increased morbidity, and mortality. Mitigating the effects of these complications requires precise and tailored management strategies.

Atelectasis, a leading cause of postoperative hypoxemia, often occurs within the first 24 hours after invasive cardiac procedures. It is closely linked to factors such as the effects of general anesthesia, inadequate postoperative ventilation, and reduced lung expansion. Effective interventions, including physiotherapy and noninvasive ventilation, have shown promise in reducing its incidence and severity.

Similarly, pleural effusion is prevalent following coronary artery bypass grafting (CABG), with most cases resolving spontaneously. However, a subset of patients may develop significant effusions requiring intervention, especially those with associated post-pericardiotomy syndrome or retained blood syndrome.

M. Al Shawabkeh (✉)
Otolaryngology Department, Ambulatory Care Center, Hamad Medical Corporation, Doha, Qatar

M. Elmestekawy
Faculty of Medicine, Ottawa University, Ottawa, Canada

A. N. Shallik
Royal College of Surgeons in Ireland Medical University of Bahrain, Manamah, Bahrain

E. Elmistekawy, N. A. Shallik (eds.), *Perioperative Care of Cardiac Surgery Patients*, https://doi.org/10.1007/978-3-032-09817-7_11

ARDS, a severe complication with a high mortality rate, is often triggered by the inflammatory response to cardiopulmonary bypass (CPB) or blood product transfusions. Recent evidence suggests that lung-protective ventilation strategies can help reduce its occurrence.

Pneumonia remains a significant healthcare-associated infection after cardiac surgery, particularly in patients with preexisting comorbidities or prolonged mechanical ventilation. Preventive measures, including perioperative prophylaxis and early ambulation, are essential for reducing its impact.

Phrenic nerve injury and diaphragmatic dysfunction, often associated with internal mammary artery (IMA) harvesting or hypothermic techniques, can lead to substantial respiratory compromise. Early diagnosis and management are critical to minimize complications.

Lastly, pneumothorax, though less common, poses unique challenges, particularly in minimally invasive cardiac surgery. Ensuring proper chest tube placement and close monitoring post-removal are essential preventive strategies.

The Pulmonary Artery Catheter (PAC) is a vital tool used for diagnosing and monitoring heart and pulmonary conditions by providing hemodynamic data. It is inserted into a central vein and advanced through the heart into the pulmonary artery, the PAC is critical in evaluating conditions like pulmonary hypertension, shock, and cardiac tamponade. However, its use carries potential risks, including pulmonary complications, infections, and thromboembolism.

Transfusion-Related Acute Lung Injury (TRALI) is a serious complication of blood transfusion, characterized by the rapid development of pulmonary infiltrates and hypoxia within 6 hours of transfusion. It remains a leading cause of transfusion-related morbidity and mortality, particularly in high-risk settings like cardiac surgery.

This chapter explores the etiology, risk factors, clinical presentations, and management strategies for the afformentioned complications, with a focus on evidence-based approaches to optimize patient care following cardiac surgery.

2 Atelectasis Following Cardiac Procedures

Atelectasis is recognized as one of the primary contributors to hypoxemia in the postoperative period following cardiac procedures; its prevalence is significant in this population, with studies reporting an onset as early as the first postoperative day [1]. Animal studies have further elucidated the relationship between postoperative atelectasis and intrapulmonary shunting, which may explain some of the hypoxemia observed after cardiac surgery. These findings emphasize the critical need for targeted interventions to address atelectasis and its impact on postoperative pulmonary function in this vulnerable patient population [1].

2.1 Etiology of Atelectasis

The development of atelectasis in the context of cardiac surgery is multifactorial, involving both intraoperative and postoperative mechanisms. During surgery, anesthesia induction and manual lung compression often lead to alveolar collapse. Postoperatively, factors such as impaired coughing, shallow breathing secondary to pain, sedation, or mechanical ventilation exacerbate these complications. By hindering effective alveolar expansion, these challenges allow the persistence and progression of atelectasis [1].

2.2 Interventions to Prevent and Treat Atelectasis

Several strategies have been explored to prevent and mitigate atelectasis in postoperative cardiac surgery patients. One such approach is the use of positive airway pressure (PAP) therapy combined with chest physiotherapy. A randomized controlled trial demonstrated that patients receiving this intervention had significantly lower radiological atelectasis scores compared to those who did not, demonstrating the efficacy of combining physical and respiratory therapies in promoting lung re-expansion [2].

Structured deep-breathing exercises have also been shown to play a crucial role in reducing atelectasis. A prospective randomized trial found that patients who engaged in these exercises had smaller areas of atelectasis and improved pulmonary function compared to those who did not engage in such exercises [3].

Noninvasive ventilation (NIV) and high-flow nasal cannula (HFNC) therapy are additional measures that have proven effective in reducing atelectasis and improving pulmonary outcomes. NIV delivers positive pressure to the airways, aiding in alveolar recruitment and preventing collapse. HFNC, on the other hand, provides heated and humidified oxygen at high flow rates, which can reduce dead space, improve oxygenation, and support alveolar stability. Both modalities are well-tolerated and have been associated with improved postoperative recovery in cardiac surgery patients [4].

Atelectasis remains a significant challenge in the postoperative management of cardiac surgery patients. Its multifactorial etiology—ranging from intraoperative factors such as lung compression and anesthesia to postoperative issues like impaired coughing and pain—underscores the complexity of its prevention and treatment. However, evidence-based interventions such as PAP therapy, deep-breathing exercises, and the use of NIV or HFNC have shown substantial efficacy in reducing atelectasis and improving pulmonary outcomes. A multidisciplinary approach, combined with continued research and innovation, is essential in addressing this common yet impactful complication, ultimately enhancing the recovery and quality of life for patients undergoing cardiac procedures. Continued research into the underlying mechanisms of atelectasis and its impact on postoperative outcomes will be instrumental in shaping future clinical practices.

2.3 Pleural Effusion After CABG Procedures

Pleural effusion is a common complication following CABG, affecting approximately 40% of patients. In most cases, these effusions resolve spontaneously without the need for intervention. However, about 10% of patients develop pleural effusions that occupy more than 25% of the hemithorax, often resulting in symptoms such as dyspnea. Other symptoms, such as chest pain and fever, are less common [5].

2.4 Classification of Pleural Effusion

Pleural effusions after CABG can be classified into early and late presentations based on the timing of onset. Early effusions typically occur within the first 15 days postoperatively and are characterized by a hemorrhagic nature with a predominance of neutrophils. In contrast, late effusions are more commonly lymphocytic in composition. Early recognition and differentiation between these types are critical for appropriate management [4].

2.5 Epidemiology and Risk Factors

Pleural effusion is the second most common reason for readmission following CABG procedures [4]. The incidence is notably higher in patients undergoing CABG involving the use of IMAs, likely due to their proximity to the pleural cavity [6]. Additionally, pleural effusion can manifest as part of post-pericardiotomy syndrome, typically developing during the second or third postoperative week. This syndrome is considered an autoimmune condition and is characterized by pleural effusion alongside other symptoms such as fever, pericardial or pleuritic chest pain, pericardial or pleural friction rub, and elevated C-reactive protein levels. Diagnosis requires at least two of these clinical features [7].

2.6 Clinical Management

Management of pleural effusion depends on its nature and severity. In cases of post-pericardiotomy syndrome, treatment often involves the use of nonsteroidal anti-inflammatory drugs (NSAIDs) and colchicine to address the underlying inflammatory process. B loody pleural effusions may require repeated thoracentesis (typically two to three procedures) to evacuate the accumulated blood. Non-bloody pleural effusions are often more challenging to treat and may necessitate the use of anti-inflammatory agents or intrapleural injection of sclerosing agents to prevent fluid recurrence [8].

2.7 Complications

In some cases, incomplete drainage of a bloody pleural effusion can result in retained blood syndrome, a condition that has been linked to the development of atrial fibrillation and an increased risk of infection. This underscores the importance of timely and effective management of pleural effusions to prevent complications [9].

2.8 Conclusion

Pleural effusion is a significant postoperative complication of CABG, with varying presentations and implications. While most cases resolve spontaneously, a subset of patients may require targeted interventions to manage symptoms and prevent complications. Understanding the classification, risk factors, and management options is critical for improving patient care and reducing the burden of this condition in the postoperative setting.

3 ARDS and Cardiac Surgery

ARDS is a significant complication associated with cardiac surgery, with reported mortality rates reaching as high as 80%. Various patient-specific and procedural factors contribute to the increased risk of ARDS in this population. Identified independent risk factors include advanced age, liver cirrhosis, massive blood transfusion, and tricuspid valve replacement [10]. Additional risk factors encompass a history of chronic obstructive pulmonary disease (COPD), current or recent smoking, prior cardiac surgery, and New York Heart Association (NYHA) class III or IV congestive heart failure [4].

3.1 Pathophysiology of ARDS Post-Cardiac Surgery

Several mechanisms can explain the increased susceptibility to ARDS following cardiac surgery. The use of cardiopulmonary bypass (CPB) is a key contributor, as it can trigger the release of pro-inflammatory mediators that initiate a systemic inflammatory response. This cascade of events can lead to endothelial damage, increased vascular permeability, and subsequent pulmonary edema, all of which are hallmark features of ARDS [11].

Wasowicz et al. conducted a study to investigate the impact of CPB on lung tissue. Lung biopsies from 20 patients, obtained 20 minutes after CPB cessation, revealed evidence of acute lung injury. Findings included extravasated erythrocytes and neutrophils within the alveoli, as well as swelling of Type I pneumocytes and endothelial cells. These pathological changes underscore the direct impact of CPB on pulmonary integrity [12].

Beyond CPB, other perioperative factors contribute to the development of ARDS. These include the body's immunological response to blood products and the effects of hypothermia, both of which can exacerbate pulmonary inflammation and compromise alveolar function. These multifactorial etiologies highlight the complexity of ARDS pathogenesis in the cardiac surgery setting [4].

3.2 Prevention and Management Strategies

Recent evidence emphasizes the importance of intraoperative lung-protective ventilation strategies in reducing the incidence of ARDS and related complications. These protocols prioritize maintaining a tidal volume of less than 8 mL/kg of ideal body weight, ensuring a positive end-expiratory pressure (PEEP) of at least 5 cm H_2O, and actively managing driving pressure. Driving pressure, calculated as the difference between peak inspiratory pressure and PEEP, serves as a surrogate marker for lung compliance. Studies indicate that keeping driving pressure below 16 cm H_2O is associated with improved pulmonary outcomes [4, 13].

3.3 Conclusion

ARDS remains a critical challenge in patients undergoing cardiac surgery, with a complex interplay of risk factors and pathophysiological mechanisms. While cardiopulmonary bypass is a significant contributor, other factors such as blood product reactions and hypothermia also play important roles. The adoption of intraoperative lung-protective ventilation protocols has shown promise in reducing ARDS incidence, marking a step forward in perioperative care. Continued research and innovation are essential to improving outcomes for these vulnerable patients.

4 Pneumonia After Cardiac Surgery

Pneumonia is a significant healthcare-associated infection (HAI) that can adversely affect outcomes following cardiac surgery. This complication not only prolongs recovery time but also increases the risk of morbidity and mortality in postoperative patients. Various factors contribute to the development of pneumonia in this setting, necessitating a comprehensive understanding of its risk factors, causative organisms, and preventive strategies.

4.1 Risk Factors for Postoperative Pneumonia

Several preoperative and intraoperative factors increase the likelihood of pneumonia after cardiac procedures. Patients with COPD, heart failure, or advanced age are particularly vulnerable due to impaired pulmonary reserve and reduced immune function. CPB further exacerbates the risk by triggering an inflammatory response and compromising lung integrity. Prolonged mechanical ventilation is another critical risk factor, as it increases exposure to potential pathogens and predisposes to ventilator-associated pneumonia (VAP) [14].

Conversely, certain perioperative measures have been shown to reduce the risk of postoperative pneumonia. The use of second-generation cephalosporins for surgical prophylaxis has demonstrated efficacy in preventing infections. Additionally, strategies such as limiting ventilation time to less than 24 hours, avoiding the use of nasogastric tubes, minimizing transfusions of packed red blood cells, and administering platelet transfusions have all been associated with decreased pneumonia rates. These findings highlight the importance of optimizing perioperative care to mitigate infection risk [14].

4.2 Microbiology of Postoperative Pneumonia

The most commonly identified organisms in cases of postoperative pneumonia include *Pseudomonas aeruginosa*, *Klebsiella pneumoniae*, and *Enterobacter cloacae*, in order of frequency. Effective management of pneumonia requires timely identification of the causative organism and appropriate antimicrobial therapy, guided by local antibiograms and resistance patterns [4].

4.3 Preventive Measures

Preventing pneumonia after cardiac surgery requires a multifaceted approach that combines evidence-based medical practices with patient-centered care. Key measures include:

1. *Elevating the Head of the Bed*: Keeping the bed elevated to at least 30–45 degrees reduces the risk of aspiration, a common precursor to pneumonia in bedridden patients.
2. *Early Ambulation*: Encouraging early mobilization after surgery helps improve lung expansion and reduces the risk of pulmonary complications.
3. *Deep Breathing and Incentive Spirometry*: Promoting the use of deep-breathing exercises and incentive spirometry enhances alveolar recruitment and prevents atelectasis, a precursor to pneumonia [4].

4.4 Conclusion

Pneumonia remains a prevalent and impactful complication after cardiac surgery, driven by a combination of patient-related and procedural risk factors. While pathogens such as *Pseudomonas aeruginosa* and *Klebsiella pneumoniae* are common culprits, evidence-based preventive measures—such as head-of-bed elevation, early ambulation, and incentive spirometry—can significantly reduce its incidence. Optimizing perioperative care and embracing future advancements in infection control will be critical to improving outcomes for patients undergoing cardiac procedures.

5 Phrenic Nerve Injury and Diaphragmatic Dysfunction

Observed following cardiac surgery, phrenic nerve injury and diaphragmatic dysfunction are significant complications reported in 30–75% of cases with radiographic evidence. These conditions can lead to substantial respiratory compromise, prolonging recovery and increasing morbidity [15].

5.1 Etiology of Phrenic Nerve Injury

The phrenic nerve, which innervates the diaphragm, can be damaged by various intraoperative factors. One common cause is mechanical injury during the harvesting of the IMA, a routine procedure in CABG. Additionally, the use of ice slush topical hypothermia—employed to preserve myocardial tissue— has been implicated in nerve injury. This method can lead to direct damage to the phrenic nerve or surrounding structures [15, 16].

A study investigating phrenic nerve conduction time (PNCT), measured through percutaneous stimulation in the neck, demonstrated its utility as a diagnostic tool for detecting phrenic nerve injury. Prolonged PNCT correlates with impaired nerve function, providing an objective marker for early detection [15].

5.2 Risk Factors and Mechanisms

Combining IMA harvesting with cooling mechanisms such as ice slush poses a compounded risk for phrenic nerve injury. Paradoxical diaphragm motion during spontaneous breathing, often observed in affected patients, raises suspicion of dysfunction. Other clinical signs include an elevated diaphragm on chest radiographs and a decreased vital capacity, indicative of compromised respiratory mechanics [6].

5.3 Diagnosis

The diagnosis of diaphragmatic dysfunction is primarily radiographic. Findings such as pleural effusion, atelectasis, and an elevated hemidiaphragm are characteristic. Ultrasound, particularly the comparison of intrathoracic and intra-abdominal pressures, serves as a valuable diagnostic adjunct. This noninvasive technique allows for real-time assessment of diaphragmatic motion and can help confirm dysfunction [16].

5.4 Clinical Implications

The consequences of phrenic nerve injury extend beyond diaphragmatic paralysis. Diehl et al. reported associations with pneumonia, cardiac arrest post-extubation, and prolonged mechanical ventilation. These complications underscore the importance of prompt recognition and management to mitigate adverse outcomes [16].

5.5 Management Strategies

While many patients demonstrate spontaneous recovery from diaphragmatic injury, some require more aggressive interventions. Early tracheostomy may be indicated in severe cases complicated by pulmonary issues such as atelectasis with hypoxia or pneumonia. Special consideration should be given to high-risk populations, including infants under 1 year of age and patients with bilateral phrenic nerve injury, who are particularly susceptible to long-term sequelae [16].

Rehabilitation and physical therapy focused on respiratory function can aid recovery. Noninvasive ventilation and other supportive measures may also be beneficial in managing symptoms and improving overall respiratory capacity.

5.6 Preventive Measures

Preventive strategies are critical to reducing the incidence of phrenic nerve injury and diaphragmatic dysfunction. Modifications in surgical techniques, such as minimizing mechanical trauma during IMA harvesting, and avoiding excessive use of ice slush for myocardial preservation, are essential. Employing alternative cooling methods and utilizing nerve monitoring during procedures may further enhance patient safety.

5.7 Conclusion

Phrenic nerve injury and diaphragmatic dysfunction represent significant challenges in postoperative management following cardiac surgery. Early diagnosis through imaging and PNCT, combined with targeted interventions, can improve outcomes and reduce the risk of complications. Ongoing research into preventive strategies and rehabilitation techniques will further enhance the care of patients experiencing these conditions.

6 Pneumothorax

Pneumothorax, while relatively uncommon in the context of cardiac surgery, occurs in approximately 1.4% of patients. This condition involves the presence of air within the pleural cavity, impairing lung expansion and compromising respiratory function. Recognizing the risk factors, clinical implications, and management strategies for pneumothorax is essential for optimizing postoperative outcomes [17].

6.1 Risk Factors and Causes

Certain cardiac surgeries, particularly minimally invasive procedures and those performed via mini sternotomy, carry an elevated risk for pneumothorax. These techniques involve smaller incisions and reduced access to the thoracic cavity, increasing the potential for complications [6].

Positive pressure ventilation, a standard component of intraoperative and postoperative care, is another notable risk factor. The mechanical forces applied during ventilation can result in barotrauma, particularly in patients with predisposing conditions such as COPD, interstitial lung disease, or status asthmaticus. These underlying pulmonary conditions weaken the lung parenchyma, making it more susceptible to rupture under increased pressure [6].

Recurrent pneumothorax has been reported in approximately 1.4% of cases following chest tube removal. This highlights the importance of vigilant postoperative monitoring, including routine chest X-rays, to promptly identify and address any recurrence. Ensuring complete re-expansion of the lung and the absence of residual air in the pleural space is critical before discontinuing chest drainage [6].

6.2 Preventive Techniques

Douglas et al. proposed a series of preventive measures to minimize the risk of pneumothorax during and after cardiac surgery. For unopened hemithoraces, they recommended creating a 3-cm opening in the mediastinal pleura to establish communication between the pleural space and the mediastinum. This step allows air to escape from the pleural space, preventing its accumulation. In cases where the hemithorax has been opened for IMA harvesting, a standard pleural drain is inserted to facilitate the evacuation of air and fluid. Additionally, a straight mediastinal tube is placed in its usual position without requiring extra tubes or unconventional placement. This approach ensures effective drainage and minimizes the risk of tension pneumothorax [17].

6.3 Clinical Management

When pneumothorax is identified, prompt intervention is required to prevent respiratory compromise. The initial step often involves the insertion of a chest tube to evacuate air and re-expand the lung. In cases of tension pneumothorax, immediate needle decompression followed by chest tube placement is necessary to relieve intrathoracic pressure and restore hemodynamic stability.

Close monitoring of the patient's respiratory status and serial imaging are critical to ensuring effective resolution. In some cases, particularly those involving persistent air leaks, surgical intervention may be required to repair the lung defect and prevent recurrence.

6.4 Conclusion

Pneumothorax is a rare but significant complication of cardiac surgery, with specific risk factors linked to minimally invasive techniques and positive pressure ventilation. Early recognition, preventive strategies, and prompt management are essential for mitigating its impact on patient outcomes. By adopting evidence-based practices, including the techniques described by Douglas et al., clinicians can reduce the incidence of pneumothorax and enhance postoperative care.

7 Pulmonary Artery Catheter

A PAC is a diagnostic and therapeutic device used to obtain hemodynamic data from the heart and pulmonary circulation. The catheter is inserted into a central vein, such as the femoral or jugular vein, and advanced through the right atrium and right ventricle into the pulmonary artery. This procedure is valuable for assessing various cardiovascular and pulmonary conditions [18].

7.1 Clinical Uses

PAC is employed in evaluating and managing several conditions, including:

- Pulmonary Hypertension Diagnosis: Facilitates determining the severity and etiology of pulmonary hypertension.
- Volume Status Assessment in Severe Shock: Provides critical data on fluid status and cardiac output.
- Evaluation of Cardiac Tamponade and Constrictive Pericarditis: Assists in diagnosing pericardial abnormalities.
- Assessment of Right-Sided Valvular Disease: Offers insights into diseases affecting the tricuspid and pulmonary valves.

These functions make PAC a valuable tool in critical care and cardiology, enabling precise monitoring and tailored interventions [18].

7.2 Complications

The insertion and use of a PAC are associated with several complications, which can be classified as mechanical, infectious, or vascular. Key complications include:

1. *Pulmonary Complications*:
    - Pneumothorax or Hemothorax: May result from trauma during catheter insertion [18].
    - Pulmonary Infarction: Prolonged inflation of the catheter balloon can lead to ischemic damage to lung tissue [18].
    - Pulmonary Artery Rupture: A rare but serious complication. A retrospective study by T.J. Kearney found that pulmonary artery rupture occurs in approximately 0.031% of catheter insertions [19].
2. *Infections and Thromboembolism*:
    - Catheter-related infections can lead to thromboembolism [18].
3. *Pulmonary Artery Pseudoaneurysm*:
    - This uncommon complication has a high mortality rate and may remain asymptomatic until it expands or causes life-threatening hemorrhage [20].

Proper technique during insertion and vigilant monitoring are critical to minimizing these risks.

7.3 Transfusion-Related Acute Lung Injury (TRALI)

Blood transfusion is a critical component of patient care but carries the risk of TRALI, a leading cause of transfusion-related morbidity and mortality [21]. TRALI is defined as the development of bilateral pulmonary infiltrates and hypoxia occurring within 6 hours of blood transfusion, in the absence of other identifiable causes [4].

7.4 Pathogenesis and Risk Factors of TRALI

The pathogenesis of TRALI involves the interaction of recipient predisposition, donor-derived factors, and cellular targets in the recipient's lungs. Antibodies and bioactive lipids present in stored blood products contribute to the development of TRALI. In cardiac surgery, the incidence of TRALI is notably high due to the frequent use of blood transfusions and prolonged cardiopulmonary bypass times. A case-control study identified risk factors for TRALI, including [21].

- Patient-Related Factors: Advanced age and prolonged time on cardiopulmonary bypass.
- Transfusion-Related Factors: Volume of transfused blood products, number of red blood cells stored for more than 14 days, total plasma volume transfused, and the amount of donor antibodies in the transfused plasma.

7.5 Management of TRALI

The management of TRALI focuses on immediate cessation of the transfusion and providing supportive care. Supportive measures include oxygen supplementation and, if necessary, mechanical ventilation to address hypoxemia. Early recognition and intervention are crucial to improving patient outcomes in TRALI cases [4].

References

1. Tenling A, Hachenberg T, Tydén H, Wegenius G, Hedenstierna G. Atelectasis and gas exchange after cardiac surgery. Anesthesiology. 1998;89(2):371–8. https://doi.org/10.1097/00000542-199808000-00013.
2. Baneton S, Dauvergne JE, Gouillet C, Cartron E, Volteau C, Nicolet J, Corne F, Rozec B. Effect of active physiotherapy with positive airway pressure on pulmonary atelectasis after cardiac surgery: a randomized controlled study. J Cardiothorac Vasc Anesth. 2023;37(9):1668–76. https://doi.org/10.1053/j.jvca.2023.05.043.
3. Westerdahl E, Lindmark B, Eriksson T, Friberg Ö, Hedenstierna G, Tenling A. Deep-breathing exercises reduce atelectasis and improve pulmonary function after coronary artery bypass surgery. Chest. 2005;128(5):3482–8. https://doi.org/10.1378/chest.128.5.3482.
4. Tanner TG, Colvin MO. Pulmonary complications of cardiac surgery. Lung. 2020;198(6):889–96. https://doi.org/10.1007/s00408-020-00405-7.
5. Light RW, Rogers JT, Moyers JP, Lee YCG, Rodriguez RM, Alford WC Jr, Ball SK, Burrus GR, Coltharp WH, Glassford DM Jr, Hoff SJ, Lea JW 4th, Nesbitt JC, Petracek MR, Starkey TD, Stoney WS, Tedder M. Prevalence and clinical course of pleural effusions at 30 days after coronary artery and cardiac surgery. Am J Respir Crit Care Med. 2002;166(12 Pt 1):1567–71. https://doi.org/10.1164/rccm.200203-184OC.
6. Weissman C. Pulmonary complications after cardiac surgery. Semin Cardiothorac Vasc Anesth. 2004;8(3):185–211. https://doi.org/10.1177/108925320400800303.
7. Tamarappoo BK, Klein AL. Post-pericardiotomy syndrome. Curr Cardiol Rep. 2016;18(11):116. https://doi.org/10.1007/s11886-016-0791-0.
8. Light RW, Rogers JT, Cheng D, Rodriguez RM. Large pleural effusions occurring after coronary artery bypass grafting. Ann Intern Med. 1999;130(11):891–6. https://doi.org/10.7326/0003-4819-130-11-199906010-00004.
9. Boyle EM Jr, Gillinov AM, Cohn WE, Ley SJ, Fischlein T, Perrault LP. Retained blood syndrome after cardiac surgery: a new look at an old problem. Innovations (Phila). 2015;10(5):296–303. https://doi.org/10.1097/IMI.0000000000000200.
10. Chen SW, Chang CH, Chu PH, Chen TH, Wu VCC, Huang YK, et al. Risk factor analysis of postoperative acute respiratory distress syndrome in valvular heart surgery. J Crit Care. 2016;31(1):139–43. https://doi.org/10.1016/j.jcrc.2015.11.002.
11. Laffey JG, Boylan JF, Cheng DCH. The systemic inflammatory response to cardiac surgery: implications for the anesthesiologist. Anesthesiology. 2002;97(2):215–52.

12. Wasowicz M, Sobczyński P, Biczysko W, Szulc R. Ultrastructural changes in the lung alveoli after cardiac surgical operations with the use of cardiopulmonary bypass (CPB). Pol J Pathol. 1999;50(3):189–96.
13. Lagier D, Fischer F, Fornier W, et al. A perioperative surgeon-controlled open-lung approach versus conventional protective ventilation with low positive end-expiratory pressure in cardiac surgery with cardiopulmonary bypass (PROVECS): study protocol for a randomized controlled trial. Trials. 2018; https://doi.org/10.1186/s13063-018-2967.
14. Ailawadi G, Chang HL, O'Gara PT, et al. Pneumonia after cardiac surgery: experience of the National Institutes of Health/Canadian Institutes of Health Research Cardiothoracic Surgical Trials Network. J Thorac Cardiovasc Surg. 2017;153(6):1384–1391.e3. https://doi.org/10.1016/j.jtcvs.2016.12.055.
15. Efthimiou J, Butler J, Woodham C, Benson MK, Westaby S. Diaphragm paralysis following cardiac surgery: role of phrenic nerve cold injury. Ann Thorac Surg. 1991;52(4):1005–8. https://doi.org/10.1016/0003-4975(91)91268-z.
16. Tripp HF, Bolton JW. Phrenic nerve injury following cardiac surgery: a review. J Card Surg. 1998;13(3):218–23. https://doi.org/10.1111/j.1540-8191.1998.tb01265.x.
17. Douglas JM, Spaniol S. Prevention of postoperative pneumothorax in patients undergoing cardiac surgery. Am J Surg. 2002;183(5):551–3. https://doi.org/10.1016/s0002-9610(02)00839-5.
18. Ziccardi MR, Khalid N. Pulmonary artery catheterization. In: StatPearls [Internet]. StatPearls Publishing; 2025. Retrieved August 28, 2023, from https://www.statpearls.com/.
19. Kearney TJ, Shabot MM. Pulmonary artery rupture associated with the Swan-Ganz catheter. Chest. 1995;108(5):1349–52. https://doi.org/10.1378/chest.108.5.1349.
20. Lafita V, Borge MA, Demos TC. Pulmonary artery pseudoaneurysm: etiology, presentation, diagnosis, and treatment. Semin Intervent Radiol. 2007;24(1):119–23. https://doi.org/10.1055/s-2007-971202.
21. Vlaar APJ, Hofstra JJ, Determann RM, Veelo DP, Paulus F, Kulik W, Korevaar J, de Mol BA, Koopman MMW, Porcelijn L, Binnekade JM, Vroom MB, Schultz MJ, Juffermans NP. The incidence, risk factors, and outcome of transfusion-related acute lung injury in a cohort of cardiac surgery patients: a prospective nested case-control study. Blood. 2011;117(16):4218–25. https://doi.org/10.1182/blood-2010-10-313973.

Falls in Surgical Wards

Fatima Emam and Rani Hammoud

1 Introduction

Falls are common among hospitalized patients and are considered a significant safety concern and a critical quality indicator in healthcare settings [1]. They can lead to severe injuries, prolong Hospital stay, increase healthcare costs, and, in some cases, mortality [2].

In comparison to the general population, hospitalized individuals in medical and surgical units are at a particularly high risk of falls due to complex and variable disease and risk factors [3]. The rate of falls varies across institutions and populations: The Agency for Healthcare Research and Quality estimates that 700,000 to one million patients fall annually [4]. Williams et al., 2014 reported a range between 3.67 and 6.26 falls per 1000 beds per day [2].

2 Risk Factors

2.1 Patient-Related Factors

Older adults are more vulnerable to falls. This is due to reduced muscle strength, impaired balance, impaired vision, and preexisting comorbidities. Patients postoperative are also at high risk of falls; this is related to surgical pain, incisions, blood loss, and fatigue that further impair mobility and balance, compounding the risk. In

F. Emam · R. Hammoud (✉)
Radiology Department, Hamad General Hospital – Hamad Medical Corporation, Doha, Qatar

Otolaryngology Department, Ambulatory Care Center, Hamad Medical Corporation, Doha, Qatar
e-mail: Rhammoud3@hamad.qa

E. Elmistekawy, N. A. Shallik (eds.), *Perioperative Care of Cardiac Surgery Patients*, https://doi.org/10.1007/978-3-032-09817-7_12

addition, some medications increase the risk of falls. This medication includes analgesics, sedatives, and anesthetics.

Other patient-related factors include male gender, previous history of falls, urinary incontinence, prolonged physical immobility, cognitive impairments (delirium, dementia, or confusion), and preexisting conditions such as Parkinson's disease, stroke, or orthopedic issues that make individuals more prone to falling [1–3].

2.2 Environment-Related Factors

This is related to the construction and status of hospital rooms and settings. Poor room setup, such as inadequate lighting, cluttered spaces, and improper bed heights, increases the risk of falls. In addition, badly fitted footwear, bathrooms with inadequate support systems, or wet floors are substantial hazards, especially for individuals with limited mobility [1–3].

2.3 System-Related Factor

Hospitals generally have systems that ensure patient safety and are led by nurses or direct health caregivers. Gaps or improper implementation of these systems can increase the risk of patient falls. These include delayed assistance due to an inadequate nurse-to-patient ratio, miscommunication about a patient's fall risk, and inconsistent or infrequent risk assessments [1–3].

3 Preventive Measures

3.1 Risk Assessment

Fall risk assessment is a comprehensive and systematic process designed to identify patients at risk of falling. Screening tools like the Morse Fall Scale or the Hendrich II Fall Risk Model can identify at-risk individuals these tools.

The Morse Fall Scale is quick and easy to use. It consists of six variables (history of falling, econdary diagnosis, ambulatory aid, IV therapy, type of gait, and mental status) that are assigned a numerical score for a total scoring of 125. A morse score of 45 and above makes the patient at high risk of fall. This scale has been shown to have a predictive validity and reliability [5].

The Hendrich II Fall Risk Model is also another scoring scale model that relies on different sets of variables; this includes (confusion/instability, symptomatic depression, altered elimination, dizziness, gender, use of antiepileptics or benzodiazepine, and a raising from chair test) a total score of 5 or more makes the patient at high risk of fall [6].

In addition to the risk assessment tools, a multidisciplinary approach involving physical therapists, occupational therapists, and pharmacists is essential to address individual patient risks.

3.2 Environmental Modifications

Room design should be adequately lighted and have decluttered pathways to ensure a safe environment. The availability of assistive devices such as walkers, canes, or handrails is important in minimizing falls. Additionally, clear signage, such as fall-risk wristbands or bed signs, serves as an effective visual cue to alert staff to high-risk patients, ensuring appropriate precautions are taken [3].

3.3 Patient and Staff Education

Patient awareness about the fall risk is of utter importance, patient should be provided with detailed orientation in regard to their surroundings and enviroment. Patient should also be educated about the importance of asking for assistant when needed. In addition healthcare provider should be trained on fall prevention strategies and early identification of at-risk patients [5, 6].

3.4 Systems and Protocols

Developing and creating hospital policies and clear systems is critical in preventing inpatient falls [4–7]. These policies can vary from one institution to another; however, generally, they have the same principal core. After admission, patient stratification is done for patients with low risk who follow general and universal precautions [7]. In contrast, for patients with moderate to high risk of falls, prevention strategies are followed, including creating a safe environment, regular nurse rounding, sitters, bed alarms, and non-intrusive video surveillance systems. In addition, post-fall management guidelines should include immediate assessment and incident reporting to address and prevent future occurrences [4, 7].

3.5 Management of Falls

Following a fall, an immediate response is needed to ensure patient safety. This starts with an assessment of patient injuries and notifying the physician or the health care team. Assessment includes:

1. Checking for any fractures, head trauma, or other physical harm
2. Vital signs monitoring for any signs of hypotension, hypoxia, or shock that may require urgent intervention.

3. Regular assessment of the patient's mental status for the upcoming 24 hours.
4. Review of patient medication.
5. General labs (CBC, renal and liver panel, and PTT, PT) to rule out any abnormalities.
6. Investigations such as X-rays or CT scans are required to assess the extent of injuries.

Additionally, detailed incident documentation is required. These include the time, location, and circumstances of the fall, as this will be used to further improve future preventive measures [1, 4, 7].

3.6 Post-Fall Evaluation

It is essential to conduct a root cause analysis of fall incidence and to identify the factors that led to the fall, as this information can be used to improve and create strategies to prevent its recurrence [4, 7].

Take-Home Message

- Falls in surgical wards are preventable with a proactive and multidisciplinary approach.
- Patient-specific risks, optimizing the environment, and ensuring robust communication and education, healthcare providers can significantly reduce the incidence and impact of falls.
- Continued vigilance and a commitment to quality improvement are essential to safeguarding patient safety in surgical settings.

References

1. Hill AM, Jacques A, Chandler AM, Richey PA, Mion LC, Shorr RI. In-hospital sequelae of injurious falls in 24 medical/surgical units in four hospitals in the United States. Jt Comm J Qual Patient Saf. 2019;45:91–7. [DOI] [PMC free article] [PubMed] [Google Scholar] [Ref list].
2. Williams T, Szekendi M, Thomas S. An analysis of patient falls and fall prevention programs across academic medical centers. J Nurs Care Qual. 2014;29:19–2. [DOI] [PubMed] [Google Scholar] [Ref list].
3. Xia L, Zheng Y, Lin Z, Chen P, Mei K, Zhao J, Liu Y, Song B, Gao H, Sun C, Yang H, Wang Y, Song K, Yang Y, Luan X, Wen X, Yin X, Fu A, Cai Y, Xie L, Li Y, Lu J, Wu X, Wang R, Gu Z. Gap between risk factors and prevention strategies? A nationwide survey of fall prevention among medical and surgical patients. J Adv Nurs. 2022;78(8):2472–81.
4. Currie L. Fall and injury prevention. In: Hughes RG, editor. Patient safety and quality: an evidence-based handbook for nurses. Agency for Healthcare Research and Quality (US); 2008. Chapter 10. https://www.ncbi.nlm.nih.gov/books/NBK2653/ [PubMed] [Google Scholar] [Ref list].

5. Morse JM, Morse RM, Tylko SJ. Development of a scale to identify the fall-prone patient. Can J Aging. 1989;8:366–7. Reprinted with the permission of Cambridge University Press.
6. Hendrich AL, Bender PS, Nyhuis A. Validation of the Hendrich II fall risk model: a large concurrent case/control study of hospitalized patients. Appl Nurs Res. 2003;16(1):9–21. https://doi.org/10.1053/apnr.2003.YAPNR2. Erratum in: Appl Nurs Res 2003;16(3):208.
7. Quality and Patient Safety Resources. Content last reviewed December 2022. Rockville: Agency for Healthcare Research and Quality. https://www.ahrq.gov/patient-safety/resources/index.html.

Transitioning to Home: Post-Discharge Strategies After Cardiac Surgery

Bassel Aboushawish, Noora Al-Hail, and Ihab Alzazoo

Chapter Objectives

- To understand the importance of comprehensive discharge planning in post-cardiac surgery care.
- To explore strategies for effective patient and family education to enhance self-management.
- To highlight the role of medication adherence in optimizing recovery and minimizing complications.
- To discuss lifestyle modifications, including diet, exercise, and smoking cessation, as integral parts of recovery.
- To emphasize the significance of psychosocial support and addressing mental health needs.
- To identify challenges in discharge planning and propose solutions for effective implementation.
- To explore future directions and innovations, including telemedicine and other technologies, for enhancing post-discharge care.

B. Aboushawish
Department of Anaesthesia, ICU, and Perioperative Medicine, Hamad Medical Corporation, Doha, Qatar

Department of Medical Education, Hamad Medical Corporation, Doha, Qatar

N. Al-Hail (✉)
Department of Medical Education, Hamad Medical Corporation, Doha, Qatar

Department of Otorhinolaryngology, Head and Neck Surgery (ENT), Hamad Medical Corporation, Doha, Qatar
e-mail: nalhail@hamad.qa

I. Alzazoo
Department of Anaesthesia, ICU, and Perioperative Medicine, Hamad Medical Corporation, Doha, Qatar
e-mail: ialzazoo@hamad.qa

E. Elmistekawy, N. A. Shallik (eds.), *Perioperative Care of Cardiac Surgery Patients*, https://doi.org/10.1007/978-3-032-09817-7_13

1 Introduction

An effective comprehensive discharge plan is essential for ensuring that post-cardiac surgery patients recover effectively, manage their health optimally, and avoid complications. The multidisciplinary team—comprising cardiologists, surgeons, nurses, pharmacists, dietitians, physical therapists, psychologists, and care coordinators—plays an integral role in providing holistic care, managing comorbidities, and educating both patients and their caregivers. Proper discharge planning not only promotes recovery but also contributes to reducing hospital readmissions, improving patient outcomes, and enhancing quality of life. The continued focus on patient-centered care and multidisciplinary collaboration is crucial for the long-term success of post-cardiac surgery patients [1].

2 Discharge Planning Process

The discharge planning process involves coordinated efforts by the healthcare team to prepare patients and their families for a smooth transition from the hospital to home. This includes developing individualized care plans, providing clear instructions, and arranging for follow-up care. Care coordinators play a central role in ensuring communication between all stakeholders and addressing the specific needs of each patient [2, 3].

3 Educating Patients and Families

Patient education is a fundamental aspect of discharge planning, aimed at improving self-management and ensuring adherence to postoperative care instructions. It is essential for patients to understand proper wound care, including the management of incisions, care of drains, and the identification of infection signs (e.g., erythema, purulent discharge, fever). Furthermore, patients should be educated about critical warning signs that require immediate medical attention, such as chest pain, shortness of breath, severe bleeding, or symptoms of thromboembolic events. Early identification of these complications is crucial for timely intervention and optimal recovery [4, 5].

4 Medication Management and Adherence

Medications prescribed post-cardiac surgery are central to stabilizing cardiac function, preventing complications, and supporting recovery. Anticoagulants, such as warfarin and direct oral anticoagulants (DOACs), are prescribed to mitigate the risk of thromboembolism, particularly in patients with mechanical heart valves or atrial fibrillation. Warfarin requires regular INR monitoring to balance efficacy with bleeding risks, while DOACs necessitate renal function assessments for safe dosing.

A systematic review highlights the significant reduction in thrombotic complications associated with optimized anticoagulation therapy [6–9]. Beta-blockers, such as metoprolol and carvedilol, reduce myocardial oxygen demand and control arrhythmias, particularly atrial fibrillation, which is a common postoperative complication [10]. Statins, including atorvastatin, stabilize atherosclerotic plaques and reduce inflammation, with studies demonstrating their efficacy in lowering mortality and cardiovascular events [11, 12]. Emerging research underscores the necessity of strict adherence to guideline-directed medical therapy to maximize benefits and minimize complications [13]. Medication adherence is a critical determinant of recovery success, yet studies indicate that up to 50% of patients struggle to adhere to prescribed regimens [14]. Interventions include structured education about medication benefits and potential side effects [15], simplified regimens through fixed-dose combinations [16], digital tools for real-time feedback and reminders [17], and pharmacist-led interventions [18]. Regular monitoring for side effects is integral to safe pharmacotherapy [19].

5 Lifestyle Modifications and Rehabilitation

Diet plays a significant role in the healing process and early recovery. If patients experience a loss of appetite or interest, they should be encouraged to consume a variety of small meals throughout the day, choose foods low in fat, cholesterol, sodium, and sugar, and increase fluid intake to prevent constipation. Maintaining a healthy weight and consulting with a dietitian to ensure no adverse interactions between food and medications, particularly anticoagulants like Warfarin, are also essential elements of dietary care [20]. Dietary modifications are central to recovery, with the Mediterranean diet being the gold standard for cardiovascular health. This diet emphasizes fruits, vegetables, whole grains, lean proteins, and healthy fats while minimizing sodium and trans fats [21]. Smoking cessation significantly reduces the risk of recurrent events, and comprehensive programs combining behavioral counseling and pharmacotherapy improve quit rates [22]. Stress management techniques, such as mindfulness-based stress reduction and cognitive-behavioral therapy, mitigate stress-induced cardiovascular strain [23]. Exercise-based cardiac rehabilitation programs are foundational to recovery, improving functional capacity, reducing mortality, and lowering hospital readmissions [24]. Setting achievable recovery goals enhances motivation and adherence to lifestyle modifications, supporting sustained engagement and improved outcomes [25].

6 Post-Discharge Follow-Up and Monitoring

Structured follow-ups are essential for evaluating recovery, adjusting therapies, and detecting complications. Guidelines recommend the first follow-up visit within 2 to 6 weeks post-discharge [26]. Telehealth has transformed post-discharge care, offering continuous monitoring and timely intervention capabilities. Telemonitoring devices track vital signs, such as heart rate and blood pressure, enabling healthcare providers to detect abnormalities early and provide prompt treatment. Studies demonstrate that telemonitoring reduces hospital readmissions and enhances patient engagement by empowering them to actively manage their recovery process [27]. A recent study highlighted the role of post-discharge telemonitoring in improving patient adherence and reducing 30-day readmission rates, particularly for heart failure patients [28]. In addition to telehealth, nurse-led collaborative care models have emerged as a promising approach to improving post-discharge outcomes. These models involve nurse practitioners coordinating patient care, ensuring adherence to treatment plans, and addressing concerns proactively. Research shows that such models significantly enhance self-care, functional status, and reduce rehospitalization rates, particularly in patients with complex needs [29, 30].

7 Identifying and Managing Post-Discharge Complications

Early recognition and management of post-discharge complications, such as infections, thromboembolic events, and arrhythmias, are essential. Timely interventions, supported by telemonitoring devices and routine follow-ups, reduce hospital readmissions and improve outcomes. Nurse-led care models have proven effective in addressing such challenges proactively [31–33].

8 Addressing Psychosocial and Support Needs

Post-cardiac surgery patients are at increased risk for mental health challenges, including depression, anxiety, PTSD, and social isolation. A psychosocial team—comprising psychologists or psychiatrists—provides counseling, coping strategies, and support groups to enhance recovery and quality of life. Both healthcare providers and patients view psychological care as a significant contributor to recovery in patients undergoing cardiac surgery. Studies have shown that psychological stress in the preoperative and postoperative period significantly correlates with increased complication rates, prolonged hospitalization, decreased quality of life, and increased risk of mortality [34]. For many patients, the indication for cardiac surgery may develop acutely or insidiously over several years. Regardless of the duration or indication for surgery, the experience is frightening to the patients and viewed as a major surgery with a high risk of complications, mortality, disability, and decreased quality of life, inducing significant emotional and psychological stress to patients and caregivers [35]. Psychological and emotional stress in cardiac surgery patients can present with symptoms of anxiety, depression, post-traumatic stress disorder (PTSD), profound fear of death, and increased suicidality [36]. Studies have reported variations in the predominant presentation of symptoms across groups depending on demographics, type and indication of surgery, postoperative experience, and effectiveness in identifying and addressing individual needs

[37]. Focused assessment using proper tools helps healthcare providers identify individual needs, provide support, and encourage significant improvement in patient outcomes and recovery [38]. Recent studies on the specific effects of psychological interventions have shown that psychotherapeutic interventions in heart surgery patients can effectively lessen anxiety and depression, mental distress, analgesic use, and reduce the incidence of postoperative complications. Individual psychotherapy during acute hospitalization has been found effective in alleviating anxiety for patients with myocardial infarction undergoing coronary bypass surgery. Relaxation techniques have proved beneficial in patients with associated arterial hypertension. Patients with mental comorbidities should continue to be assessed for emergent needs and receive psychotherapy and medication, along with appropriate care for their cardiac condition [39–41].

9 Challenges and Considerations

Barriers to effective discharge planning include logistical, cultural, and financial challenges, as well as poor communication and lack of role clarity within the healthcare team. Addressing these barriers requires structured frameworks, such as the IDEAL discharge model, and training programs to equip providers with the skills needed to address patient needs comprehensively [42–45]. Cardiac patients often face logistical, cultural, and financial barriers to mental health services. These include limited availability of professionals in rural areas, stigma associated with mental health, and high costs for uninsured or underinsured patients [34]. Healthcare providers must address these challenges by identifying patients at risk, offering timely referrals, and fostering collaborations between cardiac and mental health professionals. Training programs for providers ensure they can recognize and address psychological needs effectively [31, 46].

10 Future Directions and Innovations

Technological advancements, such as telemedicine, wearable devices, virtual platforms, and virtual reality (VR), are transforming post-discharge care. These innovations improve patient engagement, provide real-time monitoring, and enhance recovery experiences. Emerging care models and evidence-based practices further promise to optimize outcomes and patient satisfaction [38, 39, 47, 48].

11 Summary

Effective psychosocial support, interdisciplinary collaboration, and patient-centered innovations are essential for optimizing recovery in cardiac surgery patients. Tailored care plans, ongoing follow-up, and technological advancements ensure that physical and emotional health needs are addressed, resulting in improved outcomes and patient satisfaction. Post-discharge care following cardiac surgery is a complex but essential component of recovery. A multidisciplinary approach incorporating medication adherence, lifestyle modifications, structured follow-ups, and telehealth interventions ensures optimal outcomes. By integrating evidence-based practices and leveraging technological advancements, healthcare providers can significantly improve long-term patient well-being [34, 49, 50].

References

1. Whitaker-Brown CD, Woods SJ, Cornelius JB, Southard E, Gulati SK. Improving quality of life and decreasing readmissions in heart failure patients in a multidisciplinary transition-to-care clinic. Heart Lung. 2017;46(2):79–84.
2. Columbia Heart Surgery. Patient education and self-management strategies.
3. Columbia Heart Surgery. Dietary guidance for post-cardiac surgery recovery.
4. Westerdahl E, Bergh C, Urell C. Patient-reported physical activity, pain, and fear of movement after cardiac surgery: a descriptive cross-sectional study. Scand Cardiovasc J. 2024;58:2393311.
5. Gill E, Huda Su, Khan Fu. Post-discharge problems in cardiac surgery patients. Saudi J Nurs Health Care 2023:6(6):168–79. https://doi.org/10.36348/sjnhc.2023.v06i06.002.
6. Henke RM, Karaca Z, Jackson P, Marder WD, Wong HS. Discharge planning and hospital readmissions. Med Care Res Rev. 2017;74(3):345–68.
7. American Heart Association. Guidelines for post-discharge cardiac care; 2022.
8. European Society of Cardiology. ESC guidelines on cardiovascular disease prevention; 2021.
9. Enhanced Recovery After Surgery Society. Cardiac surgery recovery protocols; 2020.
10. Polsook R, et al. Self-management program post-CABG; 2023.
11. Takroni MA. A randomized control trial of cardiac rehabilitation programs; 2019.
12. Jonker LT, Lahr MMH, Oonk MHM, de Bock GH, van Leeuwen BL. Post-discharge Telemonitoring of Physical Activity, Vital Signs, and Patient-Reported Symptoms in Older Patients Undergoing Cancer Surgery. Ann Surg Oncol. 2021;28(11):6512–22. https://doi.org/10.1245/s10434-021-09707-3.
13. Bauer KA, Lip GYH. Overview of anticoagulant therapy. Circulation. 2019;140(12):902–11.
14. Estruch R, et al. Primary prevention of cardiovascular disease with a Mediterranean diet. N Engl J Med. 2018;378(25):e34.
15. Ponikowski P, et al. ESC guidelines for the diagnosis and treatment of acute and chronic heart failure. Eur Heart J. 2016;37(27):2129–200.
16. Anderson L, et al. Exercise-based cardiac rehabilitation for coronary heart disease. Cochrane Database Syst Rev. 2016;11:CD001800.
17. Rigotti NA, et al. Smoking cessation strategies. Lancet. 2020;389(10071):2055–66.
18. Healey JS, et al. Atrial fibrillation after cardiac surgery. Eur Heart J. 2019;40(10):814–20.
19. Granger CB, et al. Medication adherence in cardiovascular patients. JACC Review Topic. 2021;77(3):114–20.
20. Yancy CW, et al. ACC/AHA/HFSA guideline update for the management of heart failure. Circulation. 2017;136(6):e137–61.
21. Bhatt DL, et al. Antithrombotic therapy after coronary surgery. Lancet. 2019;394(10203):1477–88.
22. GBD Study Collaborators. Global burden of cardiovascular diseases. JAMA Cardiol. 2020;5(10):1194–212.
23. Tisdale RL, et al. Post-discharge telemonitoring outcomes. J Card Care. 2025;78(1):33–42.
24. Charles VS. Nurse-led collaborative health models for cardiac care. ProQuest Dissertations Publishing; 2024.
25. Allan R. Psychological treatment of cardiac patients. J Health Serv Psychol. 2019;45(2):72–8.

26. Ärzteblatt DÄG, Deutsches R. Perioperative psychological interventions in heart surgery. Deutsches Ärzteblatt; 2021.
27. Bond GY, et al. Post-traumatic stress in mothers of children having complex cardiac surgery early in life. Pediatr Cardiol. 2024;46(7):1823–32.
28. Child A, et al. Meeting the psychological needs of cardiac patients: an integrated stepped-care approach within a cardiac rehabilitation setting. Br J Cardiol. 2010;17:175–9.
29. Protogerou C, et al. Moderators of the effect of psychological interventions on depression and anxiety in cardiac surgery patients: a systematic review and meta-analysis. Behav Res Ther. 2015;73:151–64.
30. Pourafkari L, et al. The psychological effects of cardiac rehabilitation after coronary revascularization. Turk Kardiyoloji Dernegi Arsivi. 2016;44(3):228–36.
31. Linden W, Ellis AT. The psychological treatment of cardiac patients. In: Handbook of cardiovascular behavioral medicine. Springer; 2022.
32. Nasrawi D, et al. Delivery, barriers, and enablers to patient participation in inpatient cardiac rehabilitation. Aust Crit Care. 2023;36(3):420–30.
33. Mehta SR, et al. Effects of aspirin discontinuation on cardiovascular events after cardiac surgery. Lancet. 2020;395(10228):1569–78.
34. Patel PR, Bechmann S. Discharge planning. StatPearls Publishing; 2025.
35. Bucknall TK, et al. Engaging patients and families in communication across transitions of care: an integrative review. Patient Educ Couns. 2020;103(6):1104–17.
36. Wray J, et al. The impact of morbidities following pediatric cardiac surgery on family functioning and parent quality of life. Pediatr Cardiol. 2024;45(1):14–23.
37. Lapum JL, et al. Facilitators and barriers of heart surgery discharge: patients' and nurses' narrative accounts. J Cardiovasc Nurs. 2016;31(4):350.
38. Wong EL, et al. Barriers to effective discharge planning: a qualitative study investigating the perspectives of frontline healthcare professionals. BMC Health Serv Res. 2011;11(1):242.
39. Oravec N, et al. Barriers to successful discharge after cardiac surgery: a focus group study and cross-sectional survey. Semin Thorac Cardiovasc Surg. 2023;35(4):675–84.
40. Wray L, et al. Cardiac rehabilitation practitioners' views on patients' psychological needs: a qualitative study. Front Psychiatry. 2024;15:1434779.
41. Nasrawi D, Latimer S, Massey D, Gillespie BM. Delivery, barriers, and enablers to patient participation in inpatient cardiac rehabilitation following cardiac surgery: an integrative review. Aust Crit Care. 2023;36(3):420–30.
42. Protogerou C, Fleeman N, Dwan K, Richardson M, Dundar Y, Hagger MS. Moderators of the effect of psychological interventions on depression and anxiety in cardiac surgery patients: a systematic review and meta-analysis. Behav Res Ther. 2015;73:151–64.
43. Pourafkari L, Ghaffari S, Shahamfar J, Tokhmechian L, Nader ND. The psychological effects of cardiac rehabilitation after coronary revascularization. Turk Kardiyoloji Dernegi Arsivi. 2016;44(3):228–36.
44. Topham E, et al. Caregiver inclusion in IDEAL discharge teaching: implications for transitions from hospital to home. Prof Case Manag. 2022;27(4):181–93.
45. Lapum JL, Fredericks S, Liu L, et al. Facilitators and barriers of heart surgery discharge: patients' and nurses' narrative accounts. J Cardiovasc Nurs. 2016;31(4):350.
46. Singh Solorzano C, et al. Caregiver burden in informal spousal caregivers predicts psychological and physical health in patients following coronary artery bypass graft surgery. J Behav Med. 2024;47(6):1118–26.
47. Wray L, Capobianco L, Wells A. Cardiac rehabilitation practitioners' views on patients' psychological needs: a qualitative study. Front Psychiatry. 2024;15:1434779.
48. The Role of Patient Support Groups in the prevention and management of RHD. World Heart Federation.
49. Nasrawi D, et al. Delivery, barriers, and enablers to patient participation in inpatient cardiac rehabilitation following cardiac surgery: an integrative review. Aust Crit Care. 2023;36(3):420–30.
50. Mehta SR, Yusuf S, et al. Effects of aspirin discontinuation on cardiovascular events after cardiac surgery. Lancet. 2020;395(10228):1569–78.

MIX
Papier aus verantwortungsvollen Quellen
Paper from responsible sources
FSC® C105338

If you have any concerns about our products,
you can contact us on
ProductSafety@springernature.com

In case Publisher is established outside the EU,
the EU authorized representative is:
Springer Nature Customer Service Center GmbH
Europaplatz 3, 69115 Heidelberg, Germany

Printed by Libri Plureos GmbH
in Hamburg, Germany